SHORT NOTES IN MIDWIFERY

MIDWIFE'S COMPANION

NESTER KADZVITI MURIRA

Contents

Cardiac Disease in Pregnancy

Diabetes in Pregnancy

Pre-Eclampsia

Obstetric Emergencies

Anterpartum Haemorrhage

Eclampsia

Abruption Placentae

Premature Labour

Cord Prolapse

Multiple Pregnancy

The Fetal Skull

Intra Uterine Death

Labour

Vaginal Examination

Fetal Hypoxia

1.EMBRYOLOGY

This is the science of the development of a person before birth.

- An individual develops from fusion of the male gametes or reproductive cells, the **spermatozoon** and the female egg the **ovum.**
- Spermatogenesis or production of the spermatozoa occurs in the **seminiferous tubules** in the **testes.**
- The female reproductive unit, the ovum, develops from a single **Graafian follicle** in the ovary.
- Maturation of the spermatozoon and the ovum must take place in the testes and ovary respectively.

Chromosomes

- Mature ova and sperm contain 23 chromosomes each. One of these is a sex chromosome which can be X or Y.

- All ova contain an X chromosome while the sperm contain an X and a Y chromosome.
- A female baby is a result of a union between an X dominant sperm and the ovum while a male baby results from the union of a Y-bearing sperm and an ovum.

Ovulation

A mature ovum is released from the **graafian follicle** in the female ovary at ovulation.

The ovum moves from the pelvic cavity into the fallopian tubes and continues along the fallopian tube towards the uterus assisted by cilia and thin mucus in the fallopian tube.

Insemination

During a sexual act, several million sperm are released in semen into the vaginal canal on **ejaculation.**

Sperm swim in a medium of semen and cervical mucus through the cervix into the uterus.

Fertilization

At the time of ovulation cervical mucus, rich in sodium chloride, is thin and in large amounts.

- Cervical mucus forms channels, *arbo vitae* through which the sperm can swim. There is evidence that Y sperm swim faster than X sperm.
- If insemination or release of sperms occurs on the day of ovulation there are increased opportunities of one having a male child.
- Only one sperm penetrates the ovum.
- The head of the spermatozoon with a concentration in DNA in its nucleus, produces an enzyme, **hyaluronidase** penetrate the outer lining of the ovum, the **zona pellucid**a to enter the ovum while the tail drops off.
- An enzyme released during this process seals off the ovum preventing other sperms to enter.

- The sperm forms a nucleus that fuses with the nucleus of the ovum to form a single cell, **the zygote**.
- The zygote therefore contains 46 chromosomes which are composed of genes half of which are from the mother and half from the father.
- Development of a new individual starts from the time there is union between the **spermatozoon** and **the ovum**.

Cleavage and Implantation

Cell division is a repeated mitotic division which begins within a few hours after fertilization to form two, then four cells until within three days there is a spherical mass of cells the **morula.**

The embryo descends down the fallopian tube so that by the third day after fertilization, implantation into the uterus begins.

The cells divide into a hollow ball of cells, the **blastocyst.**

The outer layer of cells **trophoblasts** burrow into the endometrium to anchor the embryo and form the placenta.

The inner cell mass continues to subdivide to form a figure of eight structure with two cavities separated by a group of cells, the **embryonic disk**.

The top cavity fills with shock absorbing fluid in a sac, **the amnion.** The cells of the lower sac form the yolk sac which disappears within the second month.

The double layer of cells that form the embryonic disk form the new individual.

The upper layer of cells is called the **ectoderm** and the inner layer of cells is the **entoderm**.

A third layer of cells develops between the ectoderm and entoderm and this is the **mesoderm.**

The three layers of cells are known as the **primary germ layers** develop into different types of tissue,

histogenesis, and will form distinct body structures, organogenesis.

Ectoderm cells form the skin and the nervous system.

Mesoderm cells form the muscles, bones and connective tissue.

Entoderm cells form the epithelial tissue of the **internal organs**.

Trophoblasts differentiate into two layers,the inner layer of cells,the **cyncytiotrophoblasts.**

The outer layer of cells is the **cytotrophoblasts.**

The proliferation of the outer layer pushes trophoblasts into deciduas or endometrial layers to anchor the embryo, hence the name the anchoring villi.

Between the trophoblastic layer and the cytotrophoblast is a layer of connective tissue, the

mesoblast which lines the cavity of the blastocyst or the chorionic sac.

The trophoblasts continue to proliferate and become finger like projections termed **chorionic villi**.

In between the chorionic villi are tiny spaces, **the lacunae.** The chorionic villi continue to sink into the endometrial wall, eroding the endometrial capillaries so that maternal blood seeps into the lacunae.

The proliferating trophoblasts branch into a villous system the **chorionic frondosum** which becomes the placenta.

Within a fortnight rudimentary blood vessels and blood cells are formed in the mesoblastic layer and continues to develop and forms a capillary network within the villi.

The placenta consists of trophoblastic cells which divide and subdivide like branches of a tree arranged in about 200 units, the fetal cotyledons, arranged in lobes projecting into the lacunae.

At least 300-600mls of blood flows though the placenta per minute.

2. THE FETAL CIRCULATION

The fetus develops its own blood which does not mix with maternal blood.

The fetus produces its own red blood cells and white blood cells.

The fetus gets its nutrients and oxygen from maternal blood through the feto-placental unit by diffusion because the feal respiratory and digestive system are not functional in utero.

The fetus however swallows liquour which keeps the system patent and thickens to become meconeum.

Temporary Structures in the Fetal Circulation

The Ductus Venosus (from a vein to a vein) from the umbilical vein to the inferior vena cava.

- Carries oxygenated blood from the placenta to inferior vena cava from which it flows to the heart to be pumped to the rest of the fetal body.

- It closes and becomes a ligament after birth.

The Foramen ovale is a temporary opening between the two atria of the heart of the fetus

- It allows blood from the inferior vena cava to flow to the left side of the heart from which it is pumped to the rest of the body.
- It should close within five minutes of birth completely with increase of pressure in the heart. If it fails to close the baby's colour is dusky and the baby gets blue especially during feeding. The abnormality is corrected by surgery.

The ductus arteriosus (from an artery to an artery).

- This vessel is from the pulmonary artery to the descending aorta.
- It carries deoxygenated blood from the head and upper limbs to bypass the lungs.

The hypogastric arteries.

- The two vessels branch off from the internal iliac arteries to the umbilical cord and become the umbilical arteries when they the umbilical cord.
- They carry deoxygenated blood to the placenta for oxygenation.
- They become ligaments after birth.

3. THE PLACENTA

The normal placenta at term is disc shaped and **weighs one sixth** of the fetal weight.

The placenta **has two surfaces**, a fetal smooth surface and an irregular maternal side composed of the cotyledons.

The fetal surface of the placenta is covered by membranes, **the amnion** and **the chorion**.

Fetal blood vessels can be seen traversing it. The umbilical cord enters the placenta at the centre but sometimes it is at the edge, **battledore placenta.**

Umbilical vessels may run and subdivide before entering the placenta, **velamentous** insertion.

The membranes may be folded over the decidua, **placenta circumvallata.**

Placenta membranacea is thin and implants deep into the decidua.

Placenta succenturiata has an extra lobe or succenturiate lobe supplied by a small artery and vein which pass through the membranes. The lobe may be separated on delivery of the placenta and may be the cause of postpartum haemorrhage and infection.

Placenta accreta, occurs occasionally when the trophoblasts penetrate deep into the decidua.

Where the placenta implants deep into the myometrium, it is called **placenta increta.**

Trophoblasts can burrough through to the serous layer of the uterus, **placenta percreta.** A hysterectomy has to be performed in these three abnormal placental implantation cases.

Large tumours of the placenta are associated with polyhydramnios, antepartum haemorrhage and premature labour.

Fibrin deposits on the surface of the placenta cause villi within the area of fibrin deposition to loose contact with maternal blood and die causing **infarcts.**

Functions of the placenta

Substances move by **diffusion** from high concentration to low concentration.

Complex molecules are transported by **phargocytic** and **enzymatic** action

Respiratory function

Gaseous exchange takes place through diffusion in the intervillous space between maternal blood and fetal blood in the capillaries.

Nutrients transfer

Substances that are in high concentration in maternal blood **diffuse across** to the fetal blood and some are assisted by enzyme action

Immunology

Certain maternal **antibodies can cross over** to the fetus to give it passive immunity

Excretory functions

The feto-placental unit has an excretory function to get rid of waste products from the fetus.

Endocrine functions

The placenta **produces hormones** to sustain pregnancy and for the functional requirements of the fetus. The **placenta and the fetus work as a unit** in production and synthesis of hormones. Some of the hormones known to be produced by the feto-placental unit are: Oestrogens, Human chorionic gonadotrophins, human placental lactogen, human chorionic thyrotrophin, progesterone and androgens.

4.DIAGNOSIS OF PREGNANCY

Presumptive Signs

Amenorrhoea in a woman who has previously menstruated normally.

Amenorrhoea may occur because of hormonal imbalance, stress and debilitating illness or local conditions of the uterus.

Nausea and Vomiting otherwise commonly known as early morning sickness, occurs in more than 50% of pregnant women from the 4th week after the lat menstrual period.

Pica or preference or tolerance of certain foods is common in 95% women in the first trimester

Bladder Irritability otherwise known as the honeymoon syndrome is characterized by frequency of micturition in the first trimester.

Breasts enlargement and heaviness and tingling sensation.

The nipple increases in size.

The areola becomes darker and **Montgomery's tubercles** become prominent.

Distension of veins can be seen.

Chloasma or mask of pregnancy are skin changes typical of pregnancy.

Linea alba, the white line that runs from the centre of the pubis to the sternum, darkens and is known as **linea nigra**.

White stretch lines appear on thighs, abdomen and these darken in time as pregnancy progresses and are called **stria gravidarum**

Facial Complexion changes Some women may develop a smooth radiant skin while others may develop a rough skin with pimples.

Probable signs

The Vagina.

There is **increase of vascularity** causing a bluish discoloration of the vulva **Jacquemier's sign** observable from 8th week of pregnancy.

The vagina and cervix become soft and more distensible.

The **cervix becomes as soft as lips** from the pre-pregnant texture of the tip of the nose.

The **increased pulsation felt in the vaginal** fornices **Osiander's sign** due to increased blood flow is felt from 8th week of pregnancy.

Rise in Body Temperature remains from the time of ovulation onwards. Some women may experience **body shivers** typical of a rise in body temperature.

Immunological tests for pregnancy

Trophoblastic action causes high levels of HCG deposits in urine at least eight days after the date of the expected monthly period.

The Uterus

The uterus enlarges and **changes shape from pear** shape to **globular**.

The **embryo occupies the fundus** or the upper part of the uterus.

The uterine soufflé, a blowing sound can be heard on auscultation from 16 weeks due to increased blood supply.

A bimanual examination easily compresses the lower part of the uterus against the firmer fundus, **Hagar's sign** since the lower part of the uterus remains empty and soft.

. From 16th week onwards if the uterus is pushed forward on vaginal examination from the vaginal fornices, the pregnancy bulge can be felt to leave or bounce up the uterus then return to the examining finger. This called **Internal ballotment.**

Braxton's Hicks are painless uterine contractions felt on palpation from 16th week.

Positive signs of pregnancy

Ultra Sound Scan The pregnancy can be diagnosed on ultrasound scan from 5weeks gestation

Height of fundus From 12 weeks gestation, the pregnancy bulges from behind the symphysis pubis. There is **progressive enlargement** of the abdomen and **increase in the height of the uterine fundus**.

Faint fluttering fetal movements can be felt around 18-20 weeks in primiparous women and earlier on in multiparous women. This is called **Quickening**.

Fetal Heart Sounds can be picked by Doppler around 10weeks.

Fetal heart on auscultation can be heard after twenty weeks of gestation over the fetal back at a **rate of 120-160 beats** per minute.

Palpation of fetal parts. Fetal parts can be palpated and defined more clearly after 25weeks

Visualisation of the fetus. This is possible through ultrasound scan. 3-D scan will show the features of the unborn baby.

5.ABORTION

Abortion is **expulsion of a fetus from the uterus** before it is viable around twenty weeks of pregnancy.

Any woman can have an abortion although some women are likely to have increased possibilities of having abortion than others.

Causes of abortion

The causes of abortion can be :

- Faults of the pregnancy itself **(ovofetal causes),**
- Faults of the mother **(maternal causes)**
- Faults of the father **(paternal)** causes.
- Unknown

Ovo-Fetal causes of abortion

Abortions **that occur between 6-10 weeks** are largely **due to abnormality in the chromosomes** and formation of the fetus at the beginning of pregnancy.

Abortion can be due to defective implantation.

Maternal causes of abortion

Inadequate amounts of Human Chorionic Gonadotrophic hormone to support the pregnancy results in loss of pregnancy.

Local disorders of the genital tract such as bicornuate uterus, myomata and uterine retroversion disturb placental implantation and reduce space for fetal growth resulting in abortion.

Injury to the abdomen such as a blow on the abdomen, violent shaking of the abdomen and pelvis such as a bad fall or road traffic accident can cause abortion.

Deliberate interference with the pregnancy using various methods such as herbs, drugs and objects can induce an abortion.

Maternal diseases causing high temperature such as heavy flue, pneumonia, urinary tract infection, HIV infection, malaria, tuberculosis can cause abortion.

High levels of stress such as in bereavement, lack of social support can cause an abortion.

Drugs and other chemical substances

- **Off the counter medications** taken in early pregnancy may disturb the growth of the fetus resulting in abortion.
- **Exposure to chemicals** and high doses of radioactive substances can cause abortions.

Paternal causes of abortion

Half of the ovum's chromosomes originate from the spermatozoon.

- **Chromosomal defects** in the spermatozoa may cause an abortion.

- Structural defects, in the spermatozoa may be due to infections such as HIV result in an unhealthy fetus.

Varieties of abortion

Threatened Abortion

When a woman who is in early pregnancy starts bleeding vaginally, this may be a threatened abortion. The bleeding may or may not be accompanied by contractions.

This should not be mistaken for implantation bleeding which occurs as the trophoblasts sink into the uterine wall.

Implantation bleeding is small and bright red whereas abortion bleeding is heavy and may be accompanied by blood clots.

Threatened abortion

- The bleeding comes from a closed cervix
- Contractions are slight.

A vaginal examination **should not be done.**

- **A speculum examination** and gentle bimannual examination establishes that the client is pregnant and that the source of bleeding is inside the uterus.
- Bed rest, mild sedatives may make the client settle.

Inevitable Abortion

Where **contractions are strong** and the **cervix is open,** abortion is inevitable.

Incomplete abortion

- Parts of the products of conception are expelled.
- There are strong contractions
- The vaginal bleeding is heavy

Give intramuscular ergometrine 0.5mg and refer patient immediately for curettage of retained products of conception.

Complete Abortion

- All the products of conception are expelled.
- The uterus is empty.

Induced Criminal Abortion

Objects and drugs may be used to induce abortion

Curettage is done in incomplete abortion.

Septic Abortion

Is associated with incomplete abortion

- Infection involves myometrium and may spread to tubes and pelvic peritoneum
- Infection is usually caused by E.Coli or Clostridium Welchii
- The client has pyrexia, tarchycardia and offensive vaginal discharge.
- On examination the uterus is boggy and tender

Management

- Take high vaginal swab
- Treat with broad spectrum antibiotics
- Blood culture excludes systemic infection (septicaemia)
- Give ergometine
- Rehydrate client with plasma expanders
- 4-hourly temperature monitoring
- Hourly blood pressure and pulse
- Monitor urine output and look out for signs of renal complications
- Refer to a gynaecologist

Missed Abortion

Embryo dies and is retained in the uterus- a **carneous mole**

Refer to a gynaecologist for curretage to remove the products of conception

Habitual Abortion

When a woman has three abortions in succession, this is referred to as habitual abortion.

Causes of habitual abortion

- Uterine abnormality such as bicornuate uterus
- Cervical incompetence due to scars on the cervix
- Tumors like fibroids in the uterine lower segment, cervical polyps interfering with complete closure of the internal uterine os
- Hormonal insufficiency failing to support and sustain pregnancy

Management

The woman is advised to report to health personnel as soon as she falls pregnant.

If pregnant, this is **a high risk pregnancy**.

- **Refer client to an obstetrician** for pregnancy care.
- **A hysterogram and or a uterine scan** is done to exclude uterine abnormality and tumors and provide specific information on

the nature, site, size of tumor and abnormality.

- **A Shirodkar/cervical suture** is necessary to hold the pregnancy
- Bed rest and good diet are necessary to stabilize the pregnancy.

Advise to the couple

- **Comfortable sexual positions** and
- **Limit travel**
- **Avoiding strenuous** work.
- **Prevent infections such as STI's**
- Report signs of labour as soon as possible

Therapeutic abortion

A therapeutic abortion is done by health personnel in consultation with the client if :

- **Pregnancy puts mother at risk** e.g. cardiovascular disease, malignancy,
- Occurrence of serious hereditary diseases that is incompatible with life

- severe fetal abnormality that is not compatible with life like double-headed monster,severe hydrocephalus, anencephaly

6 .ECTOPIC PREGNANCY

Ectopic Pregnancy occurs when a woman falls pregnant but the fertilised ovum fails to move down the fallopian tube to the uterus.

Pathology

The sequence of events depend on the site of the implantation, the thickness of the area of the tube and the trophoblastic activity.

- Trophoblasts erode the capillaries supplying the area trying to anchor the fertilised ovum.
- Haemorrhage may be slight.
- A tubal abortion may occur.
- Where the ovum grows, the tube distends and the trophoblastic action further weaken the area of implantation until the tubal wall is penetrated and it bursts.

Bleeding occurs, the ovum may be extruded by peristaltic tubal movements.

Bleeding **may be concealed** causing a pelvic **haematoma** in the pouch of Douglas.

Bleeding **is heavy where the trophoblasts erode a large blood vessel**

Causes of Ectopic Gestation

Ectopic pregnancy can occur to any woman within the child bearing- age.

The aetiology is unknown.

Fertilization and implantation may take place in :

- the **abdominal cavity in less than 1%** of women,
- **in the fimbriated end of the fallopian tube, 17%,**
- in the **ampulla over 50%,**
- in the **isthmus of the tube about 25%** and in the interstitial portion of the uterus.
- Ectopic pregnancy **can also occur in the ovary.**

Likely causes are:

- **Infection** like Chlamydia, gonorrhoea narrowing or completely blocking part of the tube.
- **Adhesions** after abdominal surgery may narrow the fallopian tube increasing the incidence for ectopic gestation.
- The released ovum fails to negotiate through the narrow portion of the tube and continues to grow.

Signs and symptoms.

The client gives a history of:

- Amenorrhoea for 5-10 weeks.
- There is sharp abdominal pain on one side of the lower abdomen.
- There can be a palpable mass
- The fallopian tube may burst open causing abdominal bleeding.

- Bleeding may trickle out through the birth canal as dark blood without clots.
- The client may feel pain at the tip of the shoulder of the opposite side to where the ectopic pregnancy is.
- Vomiting and sudden fainting.

Signs of shock

- A very low blood pressure and a very rapid pulse,
- Signs of internal haemorrhage: restlessness, cold and clammy skin.

Management of Ectopic pregnancy

- The client is having internal haemorrhage. Severe bleeding and shock may lead to collapse and loss of life.
- Vital signs must be checked immediately and half hourly.
- **An ectopic pregnancy is an emergency.**

- The client requires an Iv infusion of plasma expanding fluid to replace lost fluid and prevent collapse.
- A sedative must be given for pain.
- A laparotomy must be done immediately to remove the pregnancy.
- Salpingectomy is an operation to remove the the tubal pregnancy.
- Blood is mopped out of the peritoneum and the peritoneal cavity washed with saline.
- The client is put on prophylactic antibiotics.

After an ectopic pregnancy

Clients must be informed that if the remaining tube is healthy they can have successful subsequent pregnancies.

- The client is advised on the need to give the body time to recover from the effects of the lost pregnancy before trying for another pregnancy.

- Check client's haemoglobin levels before discharging client from health facility
- Advise on diet rich in iron and folic acid
- A suitable family planning method must be discussed with the client before she leaves the health institution.
- Clients are advised to seek health care services early with the subsequent pregnancy for early diagnosis of normal implantation.

7.HYDATIDIFORM MOLE

This is deformity of fetal cell division in which a mass of vesicles fills up the uterus as a result of cystic proliferation of chorionic epithelium.

The vesicles vary in size and the embryo is absorbed.

Moles can be malignant or simple

Signs and symptoms

- Vaginal bleeding bright red or brownish from around 12weeks
- Undue enlargement of the uterus
- Pain and tenderness may be present
- No fetal movements can be felt
- No fetal parts are detected on palpation
- No fetal heart can be heard
- Excessive hyperemisis gravidarum
- High blood pressure in about 30% of women

Refer for ultrasound scan to obtain an accurate diagnosis

Diagnosis

- High levels of chorionic gonadotrophic hormone on simple pregnancy test
- Ultrasound scan confirms diagnosis

Management

Evacuation of uterus is done.

Sometimes a hysterectomy may need to be done where the chorionic villi have eroded the uterine wall

Complications

- Profuse Haemorrhage
- Sepsis following evacuation
- Erosion of the uterine wall
- Choriocarcinoma may follow a hydatidiform mole.

9.ANTENATAL CARE

This is organized health care offered to the expectant mother by health personnel before the delivery of the baby. This includes attention to physical, psychological and social problems that may interfere with the expectant mother's health or the health of the pregnancy she is carrying. Spouses as immediate carers of expectant mothers are encouraged to be active participants in antenatal care.

Objectives of Antenatal Care are to:

- Identify diseases that may affect expectant women's health and the health of the pregnancy and manage efficiently to prevent maternal and fetal morbidity and mortality.
- Inform clients about healthy behaviours that promote good health for a successful pregnancy.
- Monitor the health of the fetus throughout pregnancy.

- Create awareness in expectant parents of likely risks to both mother and fetus
- Provide relevant information to clients essential in informed decisions about the health of the mother and unborn baby
- Inform expectant parents about subsequent phases of the child bearing process such as labour and puerperium.
- Allay prevailing anxieties in expectant parents through discussion with clients.

Throughout the antenatal period

- Add value and worth to every antenatal visit by empowering the couple with as much health information as possible according to gestation to enable them to identify risks and make informed decisions.
- Treat every woman as an equal and show respect of feelings, beliefs and culture and respond with informed reassurance, and useful evidence based information.

during examination and routine procedures one has an opportunity to explore the needs of the client and provide client-centred health information.

- Use appropriate communication Models that enable holistic care of the client.
- Create good rapport and relaxed atmosphere
- Use humane approach, be pleasant, smile, listen to questions, pay attention, show empathy
- Provide evidence based information.
- Allow free discussion
- Allow participation in informed decision making; do not make decisions for your client
- Observe reactions and remarks indicative of fears and anxiety and need for more information.
- Be sensitive to women's fears and requests.

Collection of relevant history

Demographic history

Name, surname and address must be recorded clearly and spelt correctly to avoid confusion and mistaking with another client who may have one or more similarities.

Knowledge of area of residence

- This is essential in confirmation of client identity as well as assessment of health problems specific to certain areas, nutritional problems, or problems of access to services and other special needs specific to communities in your catchment areas.
- Residential information is essential for the above purposes as well as other needs such as home visits by health visitor.

Next of Kin:

- Enables identification of the client's social support system which is very important in pregnancy
- Enables identification of social determinants of certain health problems, clients with special needs, single women, divorced women, destitute clients

Age of client:

- This is important in identification of **teenage pregnancies** and planning for their care
- Helps to identify elderly primiparous clients and puts health personnel on the alert of relevant care and special needs as well as likely complications

Medical history:

- Reveals underlying medical conditions that may have a negative impact on current pregnancy e.g. epilepsy, heart disease, hypertension, diabetes, renal disease, asthma).

- In all these conditions, medication has to be adjusted by specialist in view of the pregnancy.
- The clients need close monitoring.

Surgical History:

- Reveals previous surgery that may be of note in the management of the pregnancy.

Family History:

- Identifies diseases that run in families that have an impact on the client and her unborn baby.
- Relevant tests, precautions and observations for conditions that run in family must be done and looked out for.
- Relevant tests must be done and observations made and health promotion provided where there is family history of

hypertension, haemorrhagic diseases, congenital conditions.

Present History:

This is key and essential in management of the present pregnancy

- Allergies: Must be known to prevent prescription of medication that may have a negative impact on the pregnancy

Reproductive history:

- **Previous pregnancies** and outcomes are essential to determine if client is on the high risk or low risk category
- Assist client to calculate the Expected or Estimated Date of Delivery (EDD) so that both the health personnel and the client work with same dates and reduce confusion.
  EDD Calculation: The First Day of the Last Normal Period plus Seven Days Plus Nine Months

Antenatal Procedures

- It is important to have baseline information of the client's health in early pregnancy so that the client's health can be assessed against this baseline information as pregnancy progresses.
- Vital signs must be assessed
- Inform client of essential procedures at each stage of care and explain to client the purpose of such procedures as well as consequences of lack of procedures.

Specimen Collection

- Explain why health personnel must collect specimens and how the information will be used as well as the likely correctional methods available for deficiencies and abnormalities.
- Explain the purpose of collecting the following specimens:

- FBC, Hb, Group and Xmatch, Urinalysis, HIV, Syphilis, Hormonal assays, amniotic fluid assays.

Weight and weight gain in pregnancy

Initial weight provides a baseline from which to monitor and provide relevant evidence based advice, counselling and health promotion in:

- Normal pregnancy weight gain increases gradually as the fetal weight increases and the amount of liquor increases
- Excessive weight gain is suggestive of conditions causing fluid retention such as diabetes, hypertension, cardiac disease, renal disease or simply over eating.
- Weight loss is suggestive of nutritional diseases in famine and extreme poverty, tuberculosis, HIV infection

Height

- A tall client is likely to have higher chances of carrying a pregnancy well. She **may have** a spacious pelvis and a relatively easier labour compared to a short client.
- Short clients tend to have larger babies for their pelvis associated with cephalo-pelvic disproportion mal-presentation, and obstructive labour that requires operative delivery.
- All short clients should have thorough pelvic assessment and should be delivered in a unit with access to emergency surgery.

Urinalysis

Urine testing is essential in the diagnosis of:

- Renal diseases characterised by proteinuria and blood in urine (smoky appearance), concentrated foul smelling urine
- Gestational Diabetes characterised by sweet smelling clear urine, with glucose deposits.

- Urinary tract infection characterised by large cell counts in urine, blood in urine (maybe fresh blood if infection is in bladder and urethra and visible deposits.
- In tropical environments, worm infestation are major causes of anaemia in pregnancy. (bilharziasis, tape worm, hookworm) may be found in a pregnant mother's urine.

General Examination

A **head to toe** examination must be done to identify obvious signs of ill health and deformity as well as indicators of previous disease and surgery.

- Explain what you want to do
- Explain what you are doing
- Explain what you have found
- Explain the available means of management.
- Provide relevant evidence based advice on the spot as you examine a client.

The Skin:

Assess the texture; exclude obvious skin diseases, eczema, pellagra, syphilitic rash, measles and other viral rashes like chickenpox

The head:

Inspect the hair:quality and quantity,state of scalp, exclude infestations like pediculosis

- High levels and low levels of thyroxin may cause hair to be brittle, falling of hair and receding hairline,
- Protein-calorie insuffiency in a diet and HIV infection may cause thin flawy hair.
- Persistent headaches- exclude high blood pressure, high temperature, stress, migraine, local infections

Investigate possible cause through interviewing and asking the right questions.

Provide relevant advice where diagnosis is clinically clear.

- Refer for further advice and management
- Cleanliness of hair, dandruff, lice and nits- advise on hair washing, use of shampoos, and management of infestations.
- Refer to infectious disease control.

Ears

- Assess position and exclude low set ears and possibility of congenital abnormality that runs in families
- Assess hearing. Exclude excessive wax and impacted wax

Neck

- Feel for enlarged lymph nodes suggestive of Tuberculosis, HIV infection, Upper respiratory infections and other systemic infections
- Exclude enlarged thyroid gland

Face

Assess skin texture, reassure where there is marked chloasma as it is likely to clear up after delivery.

Eyes:

The eyes must be symmetrical, if asymmetrical refer

If the client has strabismus, advise and refer to eye specialist

Induration may suggest strain in the eyes or trauma; advise and refer

Bulging eyeballs are suggestive of Grave's disease. Refer client for thyroid function tests.

Cataracts and poor eyesight, refer client to eye specialist. Discuss available services and exclude diabetes

Parlour in mucus membrane suggestive of anaemia. Advise on diet and refer for Hb check

In the case of obvious deformity, investigate cause and refer

Nose

- Investigate history of nose bleeds, allergies like hay fever, snoring
- Check for polyps

Mouth

- Check mucus membrane for parlour suggestive of anaemia-investigate possible cause such as poor diet, recent heavy bleeding.
- Advise, document and refer

Tongue:

- Check for sore tongue, parlour both suggestive of anaemia

Gums:

- Check for sores on the gums, to exclude syphilitic chancroid, Vit. C deficiency and other dietary deficiencies

Teeth:

- Check teeth colour, dental carries and cleanliness.
- Advise on healthy diet rich in calcium and magnesium
- Advise on annual dental check ups

Throat:

- Check to exclude enlarged tonsils

Chest:

Inspect chest for obvious deformity and scars suggestive of previous surgery.

- Auscultation of heart sounds, crepitations in lungs
- Feel for enlarged axillary lymph nodes

Chest back:

- Exclude scoliosis, hunchback

Arms:

- Check for symmetry,
- Check for tremors and investigate
- Exclude arthritis
- Check for clubbing of fingers

Nails:

- Exclude local infections
- Check cleanliness and quality of nails
- Exclude nutritional deficiencies in brittle and chipped nails
- Check the colour and exclude anaemia
- Advise accordingly

Legs:

- Watch the woman walk to observe for limps
- Exclude previous injury, bone disease, infections like poliomyelitis

- Check for symmetry
- Palpate for varicose veins
- Check feet for deformities, fungal infections like athlete's foot, quality of toe nails, calluses and bunions and advise accordingly
- Exclude diabetic foot features
- Advise on leg exercises to improve circulation throughout pregnancy

Obstetric examination of the abdomen

Inspection, palpation and auscultation

Inspection:

- Inspect skin texture and advise accordingly dry skin advise on lotions,
- Smooth and health encourage to maintain healthy skin care
- Explain the presence of stretch- marks, linea nigra and allay anxieties
- Scars: Enquire on cause of scars and types of operation. Exclude physical abuse

Size of the abdomen:

- Gives an indication of gestation,
- A small abdomen may suggest a small for dates fetus.
- Exclude Intra Uterine Growth Retardation causes such as malnutrition, hypertension, HIV infection.
- Exclude Intra-Uterine Death

A large abdomen is suggestive of:

- possible multiple pregnancy
- hydatidiform mole
- polyhydramnios
- Big baby

Shape: A broad abdomen is suggestive of:

- Multiple gestation,
- Loose muscles of grand-multiparous woman
- Obesity
- Hydatidiform mole
- Polyhydramnios.

- Seek a second opinion and refer for ultrasound scan verification

Stria Gravidarum or Stretch marks may suggest:

- Weight gain with current pregnancy
- A previous pregnancy striae

Abdominal Movements:

- Excessive movements spread all over the abdomen are suggestive of multiple limbs in multiple pregnancy.
- No movements at all is suggestive of hydatidiform mole, pseudocyaesis, intrauterine death.
- Refer for verification.

Palpation: There are five areas to palpate.

- **Fundal palpation:** Facing the client, ascertain the part of the fetus occupying the fundus of the uterus using both hands one on each side of the fundus.

- **Lateral palpation:** Supporting the abdomen with the palm of one hand ascertain the part of the fetus that lies on each side of the uterus, and where the fetus is facing by trying to feel for the fetal back or limbs with one palm.
- **Pelvic palpation:** Facing the client's pelvis, palpate the lower part of the abdomen with both hands, one on each side to ascertain the part of the fetus that occupies the lower part of the abdomen.
- **Pawlik's grip:** This is a gentle grip made using the thumb and index finger to feel for the presenting part just above the symphysis pubis.

- **Walking movements:** Using flattened fingers gently move the fingers in a walking movement to feel what lies across the abdomen

Relationship of the Fetus to the Uterus and Pelvis

The Lie

This is the relationship of the long axis of the fetus to the long axis of the uterus.

- The lie of the fetus should be longitudinal.
- Abnormalities like transverse lie and oblique lie may occur in prematurity and multiple pregnancy.

The attitude

This is the relationship of the fetal trunk to limbs and head.

- The normal attitude is that of flexion.
- The back is bent forward, the head is flexed with the chin resting on the chest.
- The thighs are flexed on the abdomen and the legs are cross legged on the thighs.
- Any deviation from this attitude is problematic at birth.

- Abnormalities can be that of extension of the head or military attitude. Engagement of the head into the pelvis may be delayed causing prolonged labour. Deep transverse arrest may occur causing obstructed labour.

Presentation

This is the part of the fetus that lies over the pelvic brim or the lower pole of the uterus.

- The presentation of the fetus can be vertex, brow, face, shoulder and breech.
- Shoulder and brow presentation are likely to cause obstructed labour.

The denominator

This is the part of the presentation that determines the position adopted by the fetus.

The denominator in vertex presentation is the **occiput.**

In breech presentation, the denominator is the.
sacrum.

In shoulder presentation the denominator is the
acromion process.

In face presentation the denominator is the
mentum.

Position

The position of the fetus is the relationship of the
denominator to six areas of the pelvis.

- The positions are:
  left and right anterior,
  left and right lateral, and
  left and right posterior positions of the
  pelvis.
- Anterior positions progress better in labour
  compared to posterior positions.

Presenting part

The presenting part is **the part that lies over the cervical os in labour** and is felt on digital examination.

Auscultation:

If using a Pinard fetoscope

- Place fetoscope where the back has been identified on palpation.
- Where the fetus is lying longitudinally, the fetal heart is usually felt around the maternal umbilical area
- Identify the mother's pulse and compare with that heard through the Pinard fetoscope
- One can use the Doppler to pick the fetal heart beat

Signs of a previous pregnancy

A woman who has had a previous pregnancy will have the following features:

- **Flabby breasts** and **prominent nipples** whereas a primiparous woman's breasts are firm and nipples may be flat
- **Lax abdominal muscles** and loose abdominal skin whereas a primiparous woman's abdominal muscles are firm and the skin is taught.
- **The uterus is broad and round** in a woman who has been pregnant before while it is ovoid in a primiparous woman.
- **Stria gravidarum are more marked** and silvery in early pregnancy while this feature occurs in the late second trimester in primiparous women.
- **Linea nigra** from previous pregnancy may be present while the primiparous woman has linea alba that darkens gradually and is prominent from the second trimester
- **The vulva gapes** and the labia minora project in front of the labia majora in a woman who has carried a pregnancy before

- The **perineum may have scars** whereas in a primiparous woman the perineum is firm and without scars
- The vagina is roomy while the vaginal muscles are tight in a primiparous woman
- The cervix is a slit which admits a finger or two whereas in a primiparous woman the cervix is closed tightly and can only allow a tip of the examining finger towards the end of pregnancy

10. POLYHYDRAMNIOS

This is when the amount of amniotic fluid in the amniotic sac exceeds 1500mls

Causes

Unknown but associated with:

- Monozygotic twins
- Fetal monstrosities such as anencephaly
- Imperforate oesophagus
- Diabetes in pregnancy

Acute polyhydramnios

- Occurs in second trimester
- It is sudden
- There is acute distension of the abdomen
- The abdomen is tense and difficult to palpate fetal parts
- The expectant mother feels severe abdominal pain
- The expectant mother may vomit

- Spontaneous abortion may occur

Refer the client for further management

Chronic polyhydramnios

Occurs slowly around 30weeks of gestation

Diagnosis

On Inspection

- The abdomen is large and globular on inspection
- The abdominal wall is stretched and tense

Palpation

- Palpation is difficult
- Fluid thrill can be felt from one side of abdomen to the other between palpating hands

Auscultation is difficult

- Fetal heart beat is muffled

Diagnosis

An ultrasound scan confirms the diagnosis

Effect of Polyhydramnios on Pregnancy

- The expectant mother feels dyspnoeac especially at night
- She feels abdominal discomfort
- She may have indigestion problems
- She may experience heartburn
- The expectant mother may feel constipated
- Abortion may occur

Effect of Polyhydramnios on Labour

- Polyhydramnios causes premature labour
- It causes early rupture of membranes
- The cord is likely to present or prolapse
- Polyhydramnios causes malpresentations
- The over-stretched uterus contracts poorly causing prolonged labour.
- Postpartum haemorrhage can be anticipated due to poor uterine contraction post delivery.

Oligohydramnios is diminished amniotic fluid

Associated with fetal abnormalities

11. ANTENATAL EDUCATION

Antenatal education should ideally be provided on a one to one basis as the client is examined from head to toe and on every subsequent visit. Spouses/partners must be encouraged to attend antenatal education classes for maximum support of the pregnant mother, identification of pregnancy risks and informed decision making.

The objectives of antenatal client education are to:

- Provide evidence based health information relevant to client's conditions and health problems,
- Explain simple and complex investigations and procedures like ultrasound scan, amniocentesis
- Explain pregnancy growth and other fetal monitoring procedures
- Discuss likely care based on examination findings

- Assist women to develop risk awareness throughout the child-bearing period
- Assist women to develop effective self-care skills
- Inform women and their spouses about events of labour
- Impart baby care skills to women and their spouses
- Assist clients to assimilate and recall information through provision of relevant health information leaflets.
- Identify and advise against dangerous community and housewives' beliefs and practices

Include the following information in client education according to gestation

- Early pregnancy exercises, pelvic floor muscle and leg exercises
- Early morning sickness and other early pregnancy symptoms.

- Sexually Transmitted infections including HIV
- Dangers of off the counter drugs
- Balanced diet for healthy pregnancy including five-a- day fruit and vegetables
- Discuss food availability, preferences, pica and allergies)
- Food taboos and advise
- Beliefs and practices in early pregnancy,
- Sex and relationships and advise accordingly

Approaches to Antenatal Education

Health information must be relevant to client according to client's need at specific gestation, (Client Centred, Culture Sensitive, Phase Related information (CCP Model) should be used.

- Individualised one to one approach especially for sensitive health issues specific to a client

- Small group discussion(centering) can be used to address specific health problems like diabetes, hypertension
- Large group approaches can be used in exercises
- Demonstration can be used in imparting special skills like baby care skills

IDENTIFYING RISK IN MIDWIFERY PRACTICE

Do not take chances with the clients' lives. If you have doubts or are not familiar with a situation, it is best to refer a client to an obstetrician.

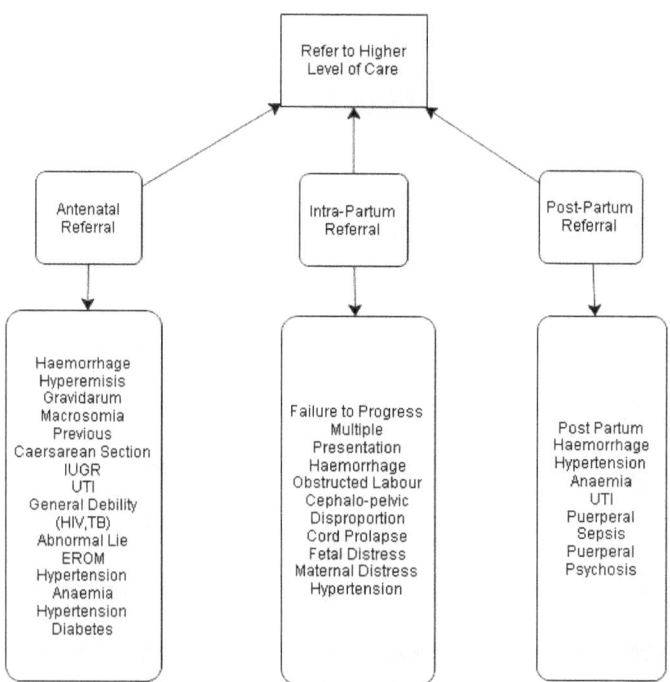

The "At Risk Clients" Refer for further management.

12. ULTRASOUND SCAN

This is a radiological investigation done for the following purposes:

- To diagnose or confirm a pregnancy (Diagnostic Scan) within the first 8 weeks after a woman has missed a normal monthly period
- To exclude ectopic pregnancy where there is discomfort in the lower abdomen in early pregnancy
- To confirm when the baby is due especially where one is not sure of when they fell pregnant (Dating Scan)
- To obtain information about the sex of the baby to enable parents to decide on names, decide on colours of clothing to buy in advance or just to know what baby they are expecting.

- To identify fetal abnormalities especially where there is excessive vomiting (hyperemisis gravidarum).
- To locate the position of the placenta in the event of bleeding in pregnancy (antepartum haemorrhage)
- To confirm multiple pregnancy and identify the number of babies in a pregnancy.
- To detect some obvious fetal abnormalities.
- To inform health personnel about the size of the baby and the position adopted by the baby in late pregnancy. This information is essential to make decisions on how the baby may be delivered.
- To see the baby's real features and not just a dark image using 3D scans especially in the last trimester
- To diagnose causes of prolonged first stage of labour and to exclude obstructed labour

13. THE SECOND TRIMESTER

- Fetal growth can be observed by monitoring increase in fundal height using palpation symphseal-fundal height and ultrasound scan.
- Exclude multiple pregnancy and polyhydramnious where the abdomen is unusually large for dates.
- Exclude Intra-uterine growth retardation (IUGR) where the abdomen is small for gestational dates
- 2nd scan can confirm sex of baby, position of placenta, fetal growth, number of fetuses and obvious fetal abnormality
- Monitor Blood Pressure closely and inform clients about signs of high BP, eclampsia, abruption placenta.
- Discuss haemorrhage in pregnancy (ante partum haemorrhage) sources of haemorrhage and appropriate action to be taken in case of this emergency

- Look for signs of anaemia, check for palor of tongue, mucus membrane of lips, conjunctiva palor, and palor of nails.
- Check haemoglobin, investigate and discuss possible causes of anaemia with client and offer appropriate advice.
- Refer anaemic clients to obstetrician for appropriate management
- Where there is excessive weight gain, undue and abnormal fundal height increase, complaints suggestive of diabetes such as (polyphargia, polyuria, polydypsia, itchy vulva), investigate for gestational diabetes

Discuss

- Possible causes of weight gain. Investigate causes and advise accordingly.
- Advise on appropriate weight loss methods especially adjustment of diet.

- Discuss appropriate diet, iron and calcium supplements for promotion of fetal growth and healthy pregnancy
- Encourage clients to drink plenty of oral fluids, to prevent urinary tract infection.
- Advise client to observe perineal hygiene especially to prevent e-coli infection.
- Advise and encourage clients to continue with appropriate exercises (walking, passive leg movements for promotion of good circulation and prevention of Deep Vein Thrombosis (DVT)
- Create awareness of signs of premature labour and prevention
- Explain the importance of rest especially in improvement of fetal health.
- Discuss common housewives tales, habits and practices in second trimester of pregnancy.

- Advise on avoidance of habits detrimental to health of mother and baby like **alcohol consumption** and **smoking.**
- Discuss beliefs and cultural practices in second trimester according to common cultural local practices in the community you serve.
- Ensure that client has relevant information and leaflets and that the client understands the information contained therein.

14. MULTIPLE PREGNANCY

Multiple pregnancy is when a woman carries more than one fetus in a single pregnancy.

Dizygotic multiple pregnancy occurs **from simultaneous fertilization** of two or more ova by two or more spermatozoa. This is chance fertilization.

- Dizygotic twins come from **two zygotes**. The ova may come from the same or different ovaries.
- **Each fetus is a separate individual** with its own placenta.
- The sex of the children may be the same or different.
- Dizygotic twins are also called **fraternal twins**. Dizygotic twins constitute at least 70 percent of twins.
- **Dizygotic twins** are more common in families with twins, in older women and multigravid women.

Monozygotic twins or uni-ovular twins.

- Monozygotic twins originate **from a single zygote** or fertilized egg.

- Monozygotic twins are also called **identical twins** or **maternal twins.** They constitute about 30 percent of twins.

- Identical twins are a result of division of a single fertilized ovum. They arise from equal division of the ovum at the inner cell mass stage.

- The fetuses **have a single placenta** and **one chorion** but each fetus has its own amniotic sac.

- One fetus may receive more nutrients than the other or one may become dehydrated and die in utero **(fetus papyraceous)**

Diagnosis of multiple pregnancy

Abdominal inspection

- The abdomen is larger than expected at the dates of gestation
- The girth of the abdomen and size of the uterus is greater than expected
- Multiple fetal movements can be seen

Palpation

- There are many fetal parts felt
- Two small fetal heads can be palpated
- Confirmation of diagnosis is through ultrasound scan

Management of pregnancy

- The client must rest more than a mother carrying a single fetus to prevent premature labor.
- The client must increase protein, iron and folic acid intake to prevent anaemia and meet the demand needs of the fetuses

Complications

- Anaemia is more common than in a single pregnancy
- Polyhydramnios is common
- Eclampsia may also occur

Labour

- Premature labour is common as the weight of the uterus weighs over the cervix
- Malpresentation is common. The frequency of presentation varies according to the size of fetuses and gestation. The babies may be Cephalic and breech
- Locked twins can occur during labour increasing the incidence of Caesarean Section
- Retained second twin may occur due to poor contractions after delivery of first twin.
- Instrumental delivery of second twin is likely due to fetal or maternal distress

- Post partum haemorrhage may occur because of the broad placental site and poor contraction of the overstretched uterus.

The Babies

- Low birth weight is common
- Each twin is usually smaller and lighter at birth than a singleton.
- Prematurity is common

15. PREMATURE LABOUR

Pregnancy lasts 280 days or nine calendar months. Onset of labour before 36 weeks of gestation is called premature labour.

Premature labour is more common in the second trimester.

Physiologically the size and weight of the fetus increase and the amount of amniotic fluid increases. These changes increase the weight of the uterus which exerts pressure on the cervix.

Other causes of premature labour

- Conditions that causes maternal high temperature such as malaria, urinary tract infection disturb the stability of the uterus which may go into contractions.
- Sexually transmitted infections like syphilis, HIV/ AIDS may cause contractions of the uterus.

- Hypertension and eclampsia interfere with placental function and the general health of the fetus.
- Abnormal uterine structure like bicornuate uterus inhibit normal growth of the pregnant uterus and its contents
- Incompetent cervix may give way to the growing fetus and increased amniotic fluid
- Uterine growths like fibroids may reduce the size of the uterine cavity and cause the uterus to go into contractions disturbing the pregnancy
- Anaemia may cause premature labour as low levels of haemoglobin may affect the health of the mother and the fetus
- Some fetal abnormalities maybe incompatible with life
- Early separation of the placenta from the uterine wall (Placenta praevia) causing haemorrhage may cause the uterus to go into contractions.

- Polyhydramnios increases the weight of the uterus and overstretches the uterus, features which may cause uterine contraction
- Multiple pregnancies weigh heavily on the cervix causing premature dilatation of the cervix
- Hormonal insufficiency or inadequate production of hormones by the feto-maternal unit may fail to support a viable pregnancy.
- Sometimes the causes of premature labour are unknown.

Management

- All expectant mothers must be informed on the first contact with health personnel in pregnancy, that premature labour is an emergency. The expectant mother must report to hospital without delay to save the pregnancy or the premature baby.

- If the woman reports to the midwife, the midwife must transfer the mother to hospital immediately!
- Exclude infections, check temperature and where temperature is high investigate the cause and commence client on appropriate treatment.
- If in a malarial area, exclude malaria by taking urgent blood slides and commencing client on treatment.
- Exclude HIV infection by doing a rapid test.
- Meanwhile put client on bed rest, left lateral position, hydrate client if dehydrated
- Reduce high temperature
- **Do not perform a vaginal examination** until client gets into hospital where a gentle speculum examination is done to assess cervical dilatation
- **Observe and record contractions**
- Be on the alert for delivery of a premature baby(have oxygen, warm incubator ready)

- Communicate with the expectant mother and inform her of possible investigations and clinical findings.

- Discuss plan of management with client.

- Inform expectant mother of the gravity of the condition and every action being taken to save pregnancy.

- Drugs that relax smooth muscle and prevent muscle spasms and contractions may be given.

- Allay anxieties.

16. ANAEMIA IN PREGNANCY

Physiological Changes in pregnancy

The blood volume increases in pregnancy to fill the vascular space created by changes in the genital system namely the changes in the myometrium and endometrium, and the development of the placenta.

The plasma volume increases gradually from the tenth week of gestation to 50% above the non-pregnant volume by the third trimester.

The red cell volume increases by 30% to meet the oxygen demand in pregnancy.

The red cell volume increase is less than the plasma volume causing a fall in the concentration of red cells in the blood and a reduction in the haemoglobin from 13.9g per 100mls in non-pregnant woman to just over 12g per 100mls from 20weeks gestation till term.

Anaemia should be considered to be present if the haemoglobin falls to 10.5g per 100mls

There is an increase in white cells and platelets.

Cardiac output increases by 30-50% in pregnancy. The heart rate increases by about 15%

The increased cardiac output is balanced by reduced peripheral resistance due to the effect of progesterone on smooth muscle.

The veins of the legs become more distensible. The pressure of the blood returning from the uterus and that caused by pregnant uterus causes a general venous pressure rise in the veins of the legs resulting in varicosity.

Causes of Anaemia in pregnancy

- Inadequate iron intake in the diet
- Excessive loss of iron due to infestations such as hookworm, malaria, bilharzias
- Infections such as HIV
- Heavy pre-pregnant menses

- Pre-pregnancy or early pregnancy haemorrhages such as extensive surgery or trauma
- Antepartum haemorrhage
- Malabsorption syndromes

Effects of anaemia on the mother

- Circulatory failure characterised by dyspnoea and tarchycardia
- Heart disease and severe debilitation
- Respiratory problems
- Prone to infections
- Poor maternal effort in second stage of labour
- Prone to Post partum haemorrhage
- Failure to breast feed successfully
- Poor healing of wounds and recovery from illness and surgery
- Increased incidences of maternal mortality

Effects of maternal anaemia on the fetus and infant

- Increased incidence of abortion
- Increased incidence of prematurity
- Low birth weight
- The infant is prone to infections

Management

- Haemoglobin must be checked on first contact with health personnel.
- Repeat haemoglobin tests at 28,32 and 36weeks of gestation
- Depending on level of anaemia and gestation, oral iron can be given where haemoglobin is around 10G
- Refer if haemoglobin is below 10g/100mls
- Refer for parenteral iron if client cannot tolerate oral iron
- Folic acid supplements may be given to all pregnant women from 20weeks gestation to meet fetal demands
- The mother is advised on a diet rich in iron and folic acid.

17. CARDIAC DISEASE IN PREGNANCY

Various changes occur in the cardio vascular system because of pregnancy.

- There is an increase of blood volume and reduction of peripheral resistance.
- The result of these changes is an increase in pulse rate and cardiac stroke volume that increases the workload of the heart.
- The blood pressure lowers

Classification of heart disease in pregnancy

Class 1. The client has no symptoms although signs of cardiac damage are present

Class 2. The client is comfortable at rest but is easily exhausted on slight effort. May become breathless and have palpitations

Class 3. Slight exertion causes dyspnoea and comfort fatigue but client comfortable at rest.

Class 4.The client has signs of heart disease even at rest.

Management

Investigate heart disease on first contact with client and refer all suspicious cases with dyspnoea, slight oedema and tarchycardia to a cardiologist.

The care of the client should aim at preventing heart failure

- Advise on reduction of daily work
- Client must rest in the afternoon and spend long hours in bed at night, at least ten hours.
- Dyspnoea must be reported immediately
- The client must be seen more frequently at least every two weeks before 28 weeks and weekly thereafter.
- Grade 3 and 4 must be admitted into hospital from 28weeks of gestation for bed rest and close monitoring.

Management in Labour

Most clients with heart disease have an easy labour and delivery.

- Nurse in an upright position
- Analgesics should be given. Avoid barbiturates as they depress respiration
- Oxygen should be given if breathless
- The second stage should be assisted delivery to quicken delivery and prevent maternal distress. Forceps may be used.

Third stage of labour

- Active management of third stage is advisable.

Puerperium

- Grade 3 and 4 should be closely monitored throughout the puerperium.
- Nurse in upright position
- Oxygen must be handy
- Prevent infection that may cause further complications like bacterial endocarditis

- Nurse in hospital for at least 7-10 days
- Advise client to keep cardiologist's appointments
- Advise on family planning preferably tubal ligation for Grade 3 and 4.
- Advise client on heart surgery

18. DIABETES IN PREGNANCY

Diabetes is a condition in which there is insufficient insulin in the circulating blood. This leads to high blood sugar levels as the body has reduced ability to convert available carbohydrates to glucose.

- The body instead burns fat to produce energy. The fat oxidation is incomplete producing **keto-acidosis.**
- In pregnancy there is a delay in the transfer of glucose from blood to tissues. High levels of glucose are therefore found in blood.
- Blood glucose levels are also increased by the presence of oestrogen and progesterone as well as human placental lactogen which oppose functions of insulin.
- Oestrogen and progesterone levels rise as pregnancy advances, insulin resistance increases as pregnancy progresses. Glucose however is readily transferred to the fetus.

Diabetes is found in about 0.2% of unsuspected pregnant women and may disappear between pregnancies.

Classification of Diabetes

Potential Diabetes

A pregnant woman has a potential for diabetes if:

- The client has a family history of diabetes
- The client has delivered a child weighing 4kg or more
- The client has delivered an unexplained stillborn child.
- The client is obese

A client has Latent Diabetes if:

- She has a normal Glucose Tolerance Test now **but**
- She has had an abnormal blood glucose test before
- The client is obese

This client is likely to develop Diabetes long after a pregnancy

Chemical Diabetes (subclinical or asymptomatic diabetes)

- The client has an abnormal GTT
- The client has no symptoms of diabetes

Clinical Diabetes

- The client has symptoms of diabetes
- The client's GTT is abnormal
- GTT is abnormal if the fasting blood glucose is 105G per 100mls

Diagnosis in pregnancy

- Urine test must be done at first contact with health personnel and in every trimester
- GTT tests must be done if client is a potential diabetic

Effect of Diabetes on Pregnancy

- Monilial and bacterial infections are increased
- The clients have an increased rate of Pre-eclampsia increasing the rate of fetal mortality
- Polyhydramnios is common
- Intrauterine death may occur as blood glucose levels rise especially in the third trimester
- There is an increased incidence of congenital malformations

Effect of pregnancy on Diabetes

- Pregnancy increases the severity of diabetes
- Intra-uterine deaths are likely to occur especially in the last trimester due to ketosis

Management

- Aim at maintaining low blood glucose throughout pregnancy.

- The client must be under the care of a physician who will decide on whether the client's blood glucose can be controlled by diet, or the client needs insulin supplementation medication.
- Where blood glucose control is difficult, clients may need to be hospitalised for stabilization.
- Where stabilization is difficult and complications are likely, delivery may be effected from as early as 32 weeks of gestation.
- Advise on diet. Refer to dietician to discuss and regulate diet.
- Client must be seen every two weeks up to 28 weeks and weekly till delivery.

Labour

- Where the diabetes is well controlled, the client may be given an opportunity to have a normal labour.

- Induction of labour is usually done at 36 weeks
- Prolonged labour must be avoided
- Caesarean section is done if fetal distress occurs

Post delivery

- Blood glucose levels must continue to be monitored.
- A small percentage of women may develop permanent diabetes post delivery
- The baby must be nursed in an intensive care unit where blood glucose levels are monitored to prevent the risk of hypoglycaemia
- The baby must be closely monitored as it is also at risk of respiratory distress because of prematurity.

19. PRE-ECLAMPSIA

This is a syndrome common in primiparous women and characterised by:

- High blood pressure
- Oedema of abdomen, sacral region, labia puffy face, legs extending down to ankles, swollen hands and especially fingers.
- Proteinuria.

The condition is common in the second trimester and rare before 24 weeks.

The actual cause is unknown

The condition is associated with:

- Multiple pregnancy
- Essential hypertension
- Diabetes
- Hydatidiform mole

Aeteology

There is vasospasm and increased resistance in the arterioles resulting in poor perfusion of the brain, liver and kidneys.

Dangers of pre-eclampsia

Maternal

- The condition may worsen and the client develops eclampsia
- Poor renal perfusion may cause renal failure
- Abruption Placenta may occur causing antepartum haemorrhage
- High blood pressure may cause cerebral haemorrhage and stroke
- If poorly managed the condition may lead to loss of life

Fetal dangers

- High blood pressure may cause placental insufficiency resulting in placental infarcts and intra-uterine growth retardation

- High blood pressure may result in decisions to deliver the baby early resulting in premature light for dates baby
- The baby may die in utero (intrauterine death)
- Due to poor intra-uterine health the baby may die after delivery (Neonatal death)

During labour

- It is likely that the baby may experience fetal distress
- High blood pressure is likely to cause Maternal distress

Management

All clients with pre-eclampsia must be referred for management by an obstetrician

- The client must be closely monitored throughout pregnancy and seen frequently for blood pressure monitoring

- The client must be advised to maintain an average weight.
- The client's weight must be closely monitored.
- The state of the oedema must be observed and client must be advised on rest.
- Advise the client to reduce salt intake in her diet to prevent fluid retention; take low carbohydrate diet to control weight gain and high protein diet to replace protein lost in urine.
- Hospitalisation may be necessary in severe pre-eclampsia.

Drugs therapy should include:

Sedatives especially at night

Antihypertensive drugs

Diuretics

Urinalysis should be done 4hourly

Monitor fluid balance strictly.

Fetal monitoring

- Ultra sound fetal growth monitoring must be done monthly
- Hormonal assays must be done for feto-placental function tests

Obstetric Management

- **Induction of labour** is done when hypertension and proteinuria persist.
- The client is delivered by 37 weeks because of placental insufficiency.
- During labour a partogram must be used to closely monitor the progress of labour and fetal well being.
- Epidural anaesthesia is preferable as it lowers blood pressure and does not affect the fetus
- Continuous fetal heart rate monitoring in labour is advisable.

- The second stage of labour must be assisted to quicken delivery, prevent maternal and fetal distress

- Third stage of labour must be actively managed.

- Post delivery the client must be sedated and close observation continued for the first 24hours.

Caesarean section can be done if:

- Hormonal assays are indicative of severe placental dysfunction

- There is severe fetal hypoxia

- Maternal condition is deteriorating or eclampsia is imminent

Characteristics of imminent eclampsia:

- There is a sharp rise in blood pressure

- The client is breathless

- There is increasingly high proteinuria

- The client's urinary output is diminished

- The client has visual disturbances like blurred vision and seeing shiny spots
- The client complains of severe headache
- The client may have epigastric pain and or may vomit
- The client gradually lapses into drowsiness
- The client may go into a convulsion

Management

- **Keep airways clear**
- Aim at preventing further convulsions give anti-convulsives intravenously and keep client well sedated.
- Aim at lowering blood pressure as soon as possible
- Deliver the client as soon as possible by Caesarean Section
- Improve renal function through infusion and diuretics
- The client should be nursed in intensive care unit until fully recovered

20. CLIENT CARE IN THIRD TRIMESTER

- Third ultra-sound scan confirms fetal growth, diagnoses fetal abnormality, fetal lie and position and decision on mode of delivery
- 3D scan shows the actual features of baby
- Inform client about investigations done and advise accordingly
- **Discuss obstetric emergencies**, antepartum haemorrhage, PIH, eclampsia, abruption placentae, premature labour and cord prolapse.
- Provide evidence based information on obstetric emergencies and appropriate action for client to take in case of emergency.
- Monitor for signs of gestational diabetes, hypertension, anaemia, heart disease and support clients with such conditions with relevant information.
- Emphasize on importance of exercise and rest and fetal health monitoring

- Discuss and practice massage and breathing in labour with couple
- Discuss the importance of sexual activity in late pregnancy and comfortable sexual positions for the mother
- Discuss and practice with client positions used in labour and child birth and advantages
- Discuss labour in detail and ensure that client preferably the couple understands the onset of labour, signs of labour, the stages of labour, procedures done in labour, analgesia in labour.
- Discuss and practice with client and spouse baby care skills.
- Ensure client has adequate post natal self-care skills.
- Ensure all clients have **emergency numbers** and sources of help to call in emergency.

- Ensure that the client has all relevant information leaflets and understands them.

OBSTETRIC EMERGENCIES

A. ANTEPARTUM HAEMORRHAGE

Haemorrhage is responsible for the highest figures of maternal mortality worldwide

"***Pregnant mothers should not bleed***".

- **Loss of blood in pregnancy is abnormal and an emergency!**
- Bleeding in antepartum haemorrhage is from both the mother and the baby

Causes of haemorrhage in pregnancy are

- Placenta praevia
- Abruption placentae
- Trauma to the genital tract
- Abortion

Placenta praevia is

When the placenta is implanted in the lower segment of the uterus. The possible causes are

- Chance implantation
- Large placenta especially in uniovular twin pregnancy
- Uterine Fibroids in the fundus
- Grand-multiparity

In placenta praevia

- Bleeding is bright red with clots
- Bleeding is spontaneous and painless

Diagnosis

Ultrasound scan is done to identify the source of bleeding, the type of placenta praevia and the state of the fetus.

Types of placenta praevia

Grade 1 The tip of the placenta is in the lower segment of the uterus. Slight bleeding may occur as the lower segment forms in the second trimester. The woman may have a normal pregnancy and labour.

Grade 2

Half the placenta lies in the lower segment. Bleeding occurs in the second trimester. The fetus may be saved but may suffer from IUGR. If the pregnancy is saved, bleeding may occur as the uterus grows and the lower segment continues to stretch. Bleeding is likely during labour. A caesarean section is the safest way to deliver the baby.

Grade 3

The placenta extends to the internal os. Massive bleeding is likely to occur at any time throughout pregnancy. The pregnancy may be lost but should the pregnancy be saved, placental insufficiency may occur and IUGR is likely to occur. The baby is best delivered by elective Caesarean section.

Grade V1

The placenta lies over the internal os. Massive bleeding is likely and the chances of fetal loss are high. If the pregnancy is saved, the client should be on bed rest. Delivery is by elective Caesarean Section.

As the placenta separates, there is reduced oxygen to the fetus. Delay in seeking help results in loss of lives.

The dangers of antepartum haemorrhage are:

a) Fetal and maternal loss

b) Shehaan's syndrome

c) Anaemia

d) IUGR

Management

- Arrange for transfer to hospital immediately!
- Put client in left lateral position

- Do not perform digital vaginal examination till client is in hospital where a speculum examination can be done
- Inform client of condition and subsequent management to reduce anxiety
- Observe for signs of shock such as rapid thready pulse, severe weakness and collapse. The mother is not in labour and therefore there is no natural control of haemorrhage by the live ligatures as experienced in labour.
- Monitor blood pressure and pulse every 10-15 minutes
- Monitor fetal heart beat every 10-15 minutes
- Put up IV fluids of plasma expanders and regulate rate according to state of the client and vital signs
- It is important to prevent infection by commencing the woman on antibiotics.

B. ABRUPTION PLACENTAE

Sudden separation of the placenta from the uterine wall in pregnancy.

- Abruption placentae can be spontaneous **but:**
- Usually follows a blow on the abdomen, road traffic accident or a fall
- It may be caused by stretching to reach for objects
- It may happen during change of position by fetus especially where there is a short cord
- It may occur where the cord is knotted or the cord has gone round the neck or the body of the fetus

Client feels

- Sudden abdominal pain as placenta separates
- The client's abdomen feels hard and board-like and tender

- Fetal movements cease

Client has

- Signs of internal haemorrhage such as rapid thready pulse, low blood pressure and gradual severe weakness
- Gasps for air and cyanosis
- Client may collapse

Management

- **This is an emergency!** Client must be rushed to hospital for resuscitation and emergency caesarean section
- Client requires IV fluids at fast rate to prevent circulatory collapse
- Caesarean section must be done immediately to save life

C.ECLAMPSIA

This is a complication of high **blood pressure** in pregnancy and is characterized by **convulsions.** Eclampsia is a serious complication that may result in renal failure, stroke or cerebral oedema as well as loss of life

- Client may have abruption placentae resulting in haemorrhage, and suffocation of fetus
- Inform next of kin/immediate carer of every step in management to allay anxiety

Management

- **This is an emergency! Call for ambulance/transport to transfer client to hospital immediately**
- Place client in a coma position
- Put up IV fluids and IV hypotensive drugs according to local policy protocol

- Check blood pressure and pulse every 10-15 minutes
- Check fetal heart every 10-15 minutes
- Check for vaginal bleeding, cervical dilatation, state of membranes and liqour
- Client is delivered by caesarean section as an emergency
- blood pressure monitoring should continue into the postnatal period

D.CORD PROLAPSE

Cord prolapsed occurs in spontaneous rapture of membranes where there is a sudden gush of liquor escapes from the uterus sweeping the umbilical cord in front of the presenting part especially where the presenting part is high up above the pelvic brim and not engaged, and where the presenting part is irregular and does not apply well to the cervix such as in breech presentation.

- The umbilical cord may fall out into the vaginal vault or it may dangle out between the expectant mother's legs
- The umbilical cord may be compressed by the presenting part causing suffocation of the unborn baby
- The cord may go into spasms once exposed to different temperatures causing fetal distress.
- The cord may pull on the placenta causing early separation of the placenta, antepartum haemorrhage, and suffocation of the unborn baby
- With reduced liquor, there is no cushion for the unborn baby anymore and this alteration of environment distresses the baby.
- **This is an emergency! Quick action is required to avoid loosing the baby!**
- Should there be delay in seeking medical help both the mother and baby are exposed to the dangers of *ascending infection*

- The client must have an emergency Caesarean section to increase the chances of a favorable pregnancy outcome

Spontaneous rapture of membranes can occur at anytime anywhere. Expectant women are advised to limit travel from the middle of the second trimester onwards.

Management

- **Call ambulance/transport to hospital without delay!**
- **Do not pack the vagina** with pads this increases chances of infection and may cause spasms of the cord.
- The expectant client must lie on the left lateral position with pillow in between legs and one pillow under the hip. Cover client's legs from hip to prevent lowering temperature.
- Inform client about the situation without causing undue anxiety

- Monitor fetal heart every 10-15 minutes
- Prepare client for emergency caesarean section

21. THE FETAL SKULL

Bones of the Fetal Skull

2 Frontal Bones

2 Parietal Bones

1 Occiput

These five bones make the **Vault** of the fetal skull

The bones of the vault are separated by membranes called **sutures**

The two frontal bones are separated by **the frontal suture**

The **saggital suture** separates the 2 parietal bones

The **frontal suture** separates the frontal bone and the parietal bones

The saggital suture, coronal sutures and the frontal suture meet at **the bregma or anterior fontanelle**.

The bregma is **diamond shaped**

It is two finger tips wide

The **lambdoidal suture** separates the parietal bones and the occiput.

The lambdoidal suture and the saggital suture meet at the **posterior fontanelle** which is one finger wide.

Sutures overlap in labour in a process called **moulding** to reduce the size of the fetal skull

Excessive moulding can occur in **premature babies**

Excessive moulding may cause **brain damage**

Excessive moulding may cause tearing of the periosteum causing **cephalo-haematoma**

14 Fused Facial Bones are immovable

The Landmarks of the Fetal Skull

Occipital Eminence

Parietal Eminence

The Bregma or anterior fontanelle

The Mentum or chin

The Diameters of the Fetal Skull

Sub-Occipito Bregmatic (SOB) 9.5cm (Vertex Presentation) Well Flexed Head. From the centre of the bregma to below the occipital prommince

Sub-Occipito Frontal (SOF) 10.0cm (Breech Presentation)(ACH) After Coming Head of Breech. From below the occipital prominence to the eminence of the frontal bone

Sub-Mento-Bregmatic (SMB) 9.5cm (Fully Extended Attitude(Face Presentation) Head Will engage when bi -parietal diameter has passed through the pelvic brim.

Occipito-Frontal (OF) 11.5cm(Face to Pubes)(POP) Persistant Occipito Posterior Military (Attitude)

Mento-Vertical (MV) 13.5cm (Brow Presentation) (Obstructed Labour) **Will not Engage**

Sub Mento-Vertical **(SMV)** 11.0cm (Face not fully extended)

Bi-Parietal Diameter 9.5cm

Bi-Temporal Diameter 8.3cm

Circumferences

SOB 29.2cm

OF 35.6cm

MV 38cm

Presentation	Fetal Skull Diameter	Length
Vertex presentation	Sub-Occipito-Bregmatic(SOB)	9.5cm
Breech A.C.H.(SOF)	Sub-Occipito Frontal	10 cm
Face To Pubes(POP)	Occipito-Frontal(OF)	11.5cm
Brow	Mento-Vertical (Will not engage)(MV)	13.5cm (Obstructed Labour)
Face	Submento-VerticalPartially flexed)(SMV)	11cm
Face(Fully Extended)	Sub-Mento Bregmatic (SMB)	9.5cm
	Bi-Parietal Diameter	9.5cm

22. THE PELVIS

The pelvis is composed **of 4bones**

Two Innominate bones on the sides and front

- Consists of the three parts, the ileum, ischium and os pubis

One Sacrum

Consists of five fused bones curved outwards and an important feature in assessment of the adequacy of the female pelvis in childbirth

It has four openings on each side through which the sacral nerves and blood vessels run.

It has **a sacral canal** the end of the vertebral canal that runs down the center of the sacrum

> The first sacral bone spreads outwards to form the **alae of the sacrum** and projects inwards to make an important landmark of the female pelvis: **The promontory of the sacrum**

One coccyx behind.

Pelvic Joints

There are **4joints**

- **2 sacro-iliac joints.**

  These are firm and immovable joints
- **The symphysis pubis**. This is a slightly movable cartilaginous joint which may give way in difficult labour
- **Sacro-coccygeal joint**. This is a movable joint and can increase the antero-posterior diameter of the outlet by moving outwards during childbirth.

Pelvic Ligaments

Sacro-iliac ligaments

Bind the sacrum and ilium at the sacro-iliac joint and are the strongest ligaments in the body.

The inter-pubic ligaments

These keep the pubic bone firm and in place

The sacro-tuberous ligaments

Stretch from the sacrum to the ischial tuberosity

The sacro-spinous ligaments

Stretch between the sacrum and the ischial spines and form the posterior wall of the pelvic outlet.

The sacro-coccygeal ligaments

From the sacrum to the coccyx

THE FEMALE or TRUE PELVIS

	Gynaecoid Pelvis	Antero-posterior	Oblique Diameter	Transverse Diameter
Anatomical Conjugate	11.5-12cm	11	12	13
Obstetric Conjugate	10.8-11cm			
Brim		12	12	12
Diagonal Conjugate	12-13cm Mean 12.5cm			
Outlet		13	12	11

THE FALSE PELVIS is the flared out dish like part of the iliac bones above the brim and has no role in obstetrics.

THE TRUE PELVIS

Is the bony canal through which the fetus must pass during childbirth.

The Brim or Inlet

Posteriorly Bound by the promontory and alae of the sacrum,

Anteriourly bound by the pubic bones

In the true pelvis, **the brim is round** except where the promontory of the sacrum projects inwards.

The diameters of the brim

Antero-posterior diameter from sacral promontory to a point 1.25cm down on the posterior surface of the symphysis pubis. It measures 11cm. This is the obstetrical conjugate

The **anatomical conjugate** is measured to the summit of the symphysis pubis and is 12cm.

The **diagonal conjugate** measured from the lower boarder of the symphysis pubis to the promontory of the sacrum is 12-13cm and measured vaginally.

The **Oblique diameters** measured from the sacro-iliac joints to the ileo-pectineal line on the opposite side and is 12cm

The **transverse diameter** measures the widest part of the brim from behind the ileo-pectineal line to the opposite side and is 13cm.

The Pelvic Cavity

Hollow curved canal from the inlet to outlet. The anterior wall is 4cm, the depth of the pubic bone

The posterior wall is 12cm the length of sacrum and coccyx.

All diameters are 12cm

The Pelvic Outlet

Upper border is at the level of the ischial spines. The bi-spinous diameter or the distance between the ischial spines is 10cm

The lower border of the outlet is diamond shaped- the pubic arch which has an angle of 90degrees anteriorly

Laterally are ischial tuberosities.

Posteriorly is the sacrum and coccyx.

The antero-posterior diameter of the outlet is from the apex of the pubic arch to the tip of the coccyx. The diameter is increased at birth as the coccyx bends backwards. The diameter is the obstetric antero-posterior diameter of the outlet and measures 13cm.

TYPES OF PELVES

Pelves are classified into **4 types** according to the shape of the brim:

Gynaecoid, Android, Anthropoid and Platypelloid Pelvis

The Android Pelvis or the male pelvis has a heart shaped brim. The cavity is deep and the outlet narrow like a funnel.

- The inter-tuberous, and ischial diameters and bi-spinous diameters are contracted.
- The sub-pubic angle and the sacro-sciatic angles are acute.
- The ischial spines are prominent.

During labour

- Posterior positions are common
- Deep transverse arrest of the head may occur
- Trauma of the pelvic floor and perineum is likely
- The second stage of labour is delayed resulting in fetal distress and instrumental delivery

The anthropoid pelvis has an oval brim.

- The transverse diameter is reduced, and is shorter than the antero-posterior diameter
- The head may engage with occiput anterior but will not rotate
- The fetal head may engage with the occiput posterior and the baby is bone face to pubes.

The Platypelloid or flat pelvis has a kidney shaped brim

It has a narrow antero-posterior diameter.

The transverse diameter is wide

The antero-posterior diameters of the cavity and outlet are also reduced

The sacrum is pushed forwards

The antero-posterior diameters of the brim cavity and outlet are reduced

Effect on Labour

- A trial of labour may be done and the outcome depends on:

  -The strength of the uterine contractions

  -The give of the pelvic joints

  -The degree of the molding of the head

- The labour is likely to be long

- The baby is likely to be born **Face to pubes**

- There are high chances of Fetal distress due to prolonged labour

- Cord prolapsed is likely to occur

- The client may require Caesarean Section

21. LABOUR

Signs of labour

Show: A thick plug of clear, jelly- like mucus is passed out through the vagina.

Show is a sign of cervical 'taking up' or effacement and opening

Labour Pain (Contractions):

- Intensified pain that starts as Braxton's Hicks start from the fundus of the uterus and move down the abdomen like a wave to sink in the groins.
- The pain is regular. It may initially be felt every thirty minutes.
- It increases in intensity as time passes.
- There is reduced time in between the pangs of pain as time passes.
- The duration of pain increases in intensity and in duration as time passes until pain

comes every 5-10 minutes and lasts up to fifty seconds.

- The pain is classified as weak contraction if it lasts up to 30seconds.
- The contractions are moderate if they last up to 40 seconds.
- Contractions are strong if they last beyond forty seconds
- Backache, a flame- like pain that intensifies on the small of the back and comes simultaneously with abdominal contraction is a common feature

Normal labour

Duration: Normal labour lasts 12-24hours.

Practical Management of Labour

Labour History taking

It is important to collect specific information about labour when a client reports in labour.

- When contractions started

- Type of pain, how long, where felt
- The state of the membranes
- If and when show was seen
- Type of vaginal discharge
- When client last ate
- When client last emptied bladder and bowels

Examination

- Vital signs: blood pressure, pulse, respirations

Abdominal Examination

This is done to assess

The shape of the abdomen which may suggest the way the fetus is lying

The presentation of the fetus that s whether the fetus is coming head first (cephalic), buttocks first (breech) or lying across the pelvic inlet(transverse lie).

The position of the fetus

VAGINAL EXAMINATION

Indications for vaginal examination are to:

- Assess the state of the vulva and report on sores, discharge, haemorrhoids, swelling
- Before investigative procedures such as Pap smear and collection of high vaginal smear in suspected infections

Vaginal examination in labour

Asceptic technique must be observed to prevent introduction of infection

The indications for vaginal examination in labour are to:

- Assess vaginal temperature to exclude infection
- To assess the type of vaginal discharge
- Establish cervical effacement or shortening
- Assess rigidity of perineal muscles

- Diagnose onset of labour by ascertaining cervical dilatation
- Assess adequacy of the pelvic cavity and outlet
- Assess cervical dilatation
- Identify the presenting part Presenting part- cephalic feels round hard mass

In vertex presentation the triangular posterior fontanelle is felt

- Exclude cord presentation and cord prolapse
- Determine descent of the presenting part in relation to the ischial spines and indicate on partogram
- Assess the state of membranes and the type of liquor or vaginal discharge
- Assess the degree of moulding and caput succedaneum and chart on partogam
- Vaginal examination –Every four hours If membranes have raptured, record time of

rapture and whether it was spontaneous rapture or artificial rapture(arm)

- Record the colour of liquor on partogram (m) for meconeum stained liquor (c) for clear liquor
- Vaginal examination is done to diagnose the cause of delay in progress of labour

Active labour is from 3cm cervical dilatation

Draw the alert line, the action and the transfer lines on partograph

Chart the following on partogram chart:

- Fetal heart rate every ½ hour
- Type of contractions should be mild to strong
- State of membranes and colour of liquour
- Analgesia given and any other drugs like antibiotics, anti-emetics,
- Augmentation of labour, that is oxytocin use amount and rate

- Blood pressure, pulse and respirations hourly
- Temperature 4hourly
- Urinary output and analysis of the urine 4hourly
- Ensure the couple is well informed about the stages of labour.
- Keep the couple informed of events at each stage.
- Share the examination results with the couple.

22.FETAL HYPOXIA

Lack of adequate amounts of oxygen to the fetus

Causes are maternal, fetal, and iatrogenic.

Maternal causes

Conditions that reduce blood floor to the placental site such as:

- anaemia,
- pre-clampsia,
- heart disease especially Grade 3 and 4,
- severe infections like malaria
- Placental dysfunction eg. Abruption placentae

Fetal causes

- Cord round the neck or limb,
- true knots in the cord,
- placental infarcts,
- cord prolapse,
- reflex brardycardia,

- cephalo-pelvic disproportion,
- prolonged labour

Iatrogenic Causes

- Drugs such as oxytocins, anaesthesia, analgesics such as Pethidine, Morphine

Diagnosis of fetal distress

- Fetal tarchycardia or heart rate of more than 160 beats
- Fetal brardycardia or heart rate below 110
- Meconeum in the liquour
- Fetal heart rate should be listened to when the contraction starts, during a contraction and after a contraction to assess the degree of distress
- Continuous fetal monitoring can be done where a fetal cardiotocogram is available
- Fetal blood sampling for fetal acidosis can also be done

Management

Fetal distress in first stage of labour

- Communicate with client about observations
- Nurse patient in an upright position
- Give the client IVI Dextrose 10% and continue infusion of 5%Dextrose
- If on oxytocin, stop the infusion
- Give oxygen
- Prepare for Caesarean section

Fetal Distress in the second stage

- Perform an episiotomy to quicken delivery
- Forceps or vacuum extraction can be done depending on expertise available
- Prepare for resuscitation of the newborn

23. PAIN RELIEF IN LABOUR

Pain relief in labour must be discussed and understood by the client during antenatal education to enable women to make an informed choice of analgesia when in labour.

The natural methods of pain relief

Warm Water

A woman can have a warm shower or soak herself in a bath as she labours. Water births have been reported to be comfortable and tolerable.al relief of pain.

Breathing

- Breathing with contractions provides a natural way of pain relief in labour.
- The pregnant woman and her spouse should be made familiar with how to breathe in labour during antenatal classes.

Sedation in early labour

- Pain threshold varies from one woman to the next. It is important to communicate with the client to understand her needs.
- Some women prefer a drug free labour.
- The client's choice must be respected.
- Barbiturates and tranquilizers can be used in early labour. Assess effectiveness of drug used through effective communication with client.
- Explain why a woman cannot access the method of analgesia she desires e.g. the stage of labour, availability of expertise etc.

Analgesics

Pethidine and Morphine have been widely used for pain relief in early labour.

Effect on the mother

- They have an analgesic effect of 2-4 hours.
- They cause drowsiness and affect maternal effort in the second stage of labour.

Effect on the infant

- They cause fetal distress
- They increase the need for fetal resuscitation.

It is important that assessment of the progress of labour is done before administration of these drugs. They should therefore be avoided in late labour from six centimetres of cervical dilatation

Inhalation Analgesia

The widely used is Nitrous Oxide. This is most useful in the late first stage and second stage of labour

- The client must be able to use it. It is important that clients are familiar with deep breathing technique.
- It has no residual effect on the mother and infant.

Epidural anaesthesia

This method of analgesia is widely used. Self-regulatory epidural is becoming popular with women.

- The client must be in established labour.
- Should operative delivery be required, it can be done without the need for additional anaesthesia.

Advantages

- It enables a painless labour and operative delivery without affecting consciousness
- It does not affect the fetus

Disadvantages

It requires an anaesthetist to administer it.

Side effects

- Causes lowering of blood pressure
- Client is confined to bed
- Client requires catheterization

- Affects maternal effort in the second stage of labour
- Increases the need for assisted delivery such as forceps delivery
- May cause headaches and residual weakness of limbs.

Para-cervical block and Pudendal nerve block are rarely used now especially with the reported advantages of the epidural.

24. MECHANISM OF LABOUR

MECHANISM OF VERTEX PRESENTATION

Flexion   With increased contractions, the head is flexed and descent takes place with increasing flexion

Internal Rotation of the Head

The occiput reaches the pelvic floor first and rotates 1/8 of a circle forwards to become anterior

Crowning

The occiput escapes under the symphysis pubis and the head is crowned

Extension

The sinciput, face and chin sweep the perineum and the head is born by a movement of externtion.

Restitution

The occiput turns 1/8 of a circle back to where it was before internal rotation and the head rights itself with the shoulders

Internal rotation of the shoulders

The anterior shoulder reaches the pelvic floor first and rotates 1/8 of a circle forwards at the same time as there is external rotation of the head.

The rest of the body is delivered by a movement of lateral flexion.

BREECH PRESENTATION

There are three classifications of breech presentation

- Breech with extended legs
- Breech with flexed legs
- Footling and knee presentations

Causes of breech presentation

- Unknown
- Associated with big babies
- Where there is a short cord the fetus tends to face the placenta
- If the placenta is situated in the body of the uterus and the lower segment

- In multiple pregnancy, one fetus may adopt a breech position
- In prematurity the fetus may adopt a breech position
- Tumours in the lower uterine segment

Diagnosis

Palpation

- The head can be palpated in the fundus
- The lie is longitudinal
- There is a large irregular soft mass on pelvic palpation and Pawlick's grip

Auscultation

- The fetal heart is heard above the umbilicus

Vaginal Examination

The breech is soft and irregular unlike the head which is round and hard

Ultrasound scan or radiology will confirm diagnosis

Mechanism of Breech Delivery

- **Engagement of the breech occurs in the oblique** or transverse diameter of the pelvic brim

- The buttocks reach the pelvic floor and internal rotation occurs.The bitrochanteric diameter lies in the antero-posterior diameter of the pelvic outlet.

- The anterior buttock appears at the vulva by lateral flexion of the trunk

- The buttocks are born while the shoulders adjust to engage in the transverse diameter of the brim. There is external rotation of the buttocks so that the back is uppermost

- The shoulders reach the pelvic floor and undergo internal rotation so that the bisachromial diameter lies in the antero-posterior diameter of the pelvic outlet. The buttocks rotate anteriorly in a movement called restitution.

- The head engages in the pelvic brim simultaneously. The saggital suture lies in the transverse diameter of the brim.
- The anterior shoulder is born from under the symphysis pubis by lateral flexion of the trunk
- On reaching the pelvic floor internal rotation occurs through 90 degrees. Further descent and further flexion occurs. The occiput lies behind the symphysis pubis.
- The chin, mouth, nose and forehead sweep the perineum

Management of labour in Breech Presentation

Attempt delivery only in emergency! **Refer all breech presentation to hospital with facility for Caesarean Section.**

- Confirm presentation through a vaginal examination
- Exclude cord prolapsed when membranes rupture

- Manage labour like any normal labour

Second stage of labour

- An episiotomy must be done as the buttocks distend the vulva

Hands off the breech! Allow the natural process of delivery where possible.

- If buttocks are not expelled, forefingers are inserted in fold of the groins and slight traction applied.
- If breech is extended the legs are released by applying pressure on the popliteal fossa outwards to abduct and flex the thighs
- Bring down the loop of the cord to prevent traction on the cord which may distress the baby

Delivery of the shoulders

- **Apply Lovset manoeuvre** to deliver shoulders by rotating the body of the baby 180 degrees so that the posterior shoulder lies anteriorly. The shoulder may be delivered spontaneously or lifted out using one finger.

- Rotate the body of the baby 180 degrees in the opposite direction to deliver the other arm which can be delivered spontaneously or can be hooked out with a finger.

Delivery of the head

- When the nape of the neck appears in the sub-pubic angle, Aim at maintaining full flexion of the head.
- Grasp the baby by the ankles and swing the baby over the vulva so that the chin and mouth appear on the vulva.
- Extract mucus from mouth and pharynx. The head may be delivered at this stage with slight supra-pubic pressure

Mauriceau – Smellie- Veit technique

- This is an alternative method for delivery of the head

- Place middle finger of left arm on the sub-occipital region.
- Place the ring and index fingers on the shoulders.
- Place the supinated right arm under the baby with the baby lying over the arm
- Place index finger in the baby's mouth and the ring and index fingers on the malar bones. This hand applies flexion and the two hands gently apply traction to the baby downwards and backwards then downward and forward to deliver the head.

Fetal Complications of breech delivery

- Cord prolapse
- Fetal distress
- Fractures of limbs
- Abruptio placenta
- Impacted shoulders
- Arrest of after coming head
- Brain injury

- Nerve injury
- Prolonged labour
- Loss of baby either as a stillbirth or neonatal death

Maternal complications

- Extensive Cervical, vaginal and perineal tears
- Haemorrhage
- Maternal distress
- Ascending Infection

25. POSITIONS USED IN LABOUR AND CHILDBIRTH

A woman in labour does not have to lye in bed, she should be active.

- In the first stage of labour, an upright position has the advantage that the fetus can descend into the pelvis assisted by gravity.
- It is easier for the presenting part to negotiate its way into the pelvis as it can follow the natural curve of the back, Curve of Carus, into the pelvis.

Positions that are encouraged in the first stage of labour are those that keep the back in an upright position such as:

- Walking about, standing, and leaning against a chair, a firm table or wall
- Leaning against one's partner is ideal for back massage which enables the partner to participate actively in the events of labour.

The partner must stand astride to be able to stand firmly and support his spouse.

- Sitting in a firm chair with a firm straight back keeps the back in an upright position and enables the fetus to descend into the pelvis following the natural curve of the spine.

- Squatting for long or short periods depending on one's tolerance also encourages decent of the fetus.

- Kneeling and leaning on cushions or pillows also keeps the back straight and encourages a fairly quick decent of the fetus into the pelvis.

- A labouring woman can sit in a warm tub of water. Warm water is a natural method of pain relief.

N.B. Ensure that women are familiar with these positions before labour starts. These positions should be practiced in the antenatal classes so that there is mutual understanding when the

woman is asked to adopt the positions in labour.

Advantages of these positions

- These positions make it easier for the labouring woman to be supported by a partner and make it easy to reach the back for massage.
- These positions have been associated with a less painful labour in which one may not need pain relief.
- There is less pressure on the blood vessels that supply the uterus with blood meaning that the fetus has a good supply of oxygen throughout the first stage of labour.
- The contractions always start from the fundus pushing downwards like a wave and being in an upright position means that the contractions work better.
- The cervical dilation is faster as the presenting part applies to the cervix better

making labour shorter. These positions have been reported to shorten labour compared to lying in bed.

- There is less maternal and fetal distress.

The second stage of labour:

- Marked by full dilatation
- Some clients may vomit
- Expulsive strong contractions lasting 60-90 seconds generally at 3-5minute intervals
- Head moves forwards with each contraction and recedes in between contractions
- Record FHR every Five minutes, with contraction and after contraction
- Note maternal state-exhaustion, dehydration
- Note vaginal discharge
- Meconeum,what type-thin put up 5%Dextrose infusion and give oxygen
- Thick meconeum may need assisted delivery- vacuum extraction, forceps delivery

to quicken delivery. Baby will require antibiotics post delivery

- Bloody vaginal discharge-could be vaginal bruising, could be ruptured varicose veins, could be abruption placentae
- ¼ hourly maternal pulse

Delivery Positions

- A woman can squat supported by pillows or by two people one on each side and delivery can be effected in that position.
- A labouring woman can sit in a birth stool These positions are more comfortable than lying down.
- Client can sit supported by pillows.

Advantages of these positions

- The second stage of labour is shortened when a woman is in an upright position.
- Perineal tears are minimal.
- Post partum haemorrhage is minimal

- The newly born baby is less stressed reducing the need for fetal resuscitation.

As presenting part distends the perineum:

- Place sanitary towel over the anus to prevent contact of faecal matter with baby
- Left hand gently assists flexion of fetal head
- Crowning-Parietal eminences are visible on the vulva
- Advise mother to pant instead of pushing to protect perineum from tearing

Episiotomy

A surgical incision made on the perineum during the perineal phase of labour

Advantages

- Prevents ragged perineal tears
- Protects rectal muscle
- It prevents pressure and injury to fetal head

- It enables quick delivery of baby in fetal distress and maternal exhaustion

Procedure

- Two fingers are placed between presenting part and perineal muscle to prevent injury of the fetus
- 5-10mls of lignocain injected into perineal muscle in a fan-like manner
- Incision is made with a contraction from medial raphe preferably medo-lateral incision
- Give syntometrine with delivery of anterior shoulder
- Feel for the cord around the neck and slip it over the head
- If cord is too tight clamp the cord and separate it between two Spencer Wells Forceps
- Ideally the cord should be cut 2.5cm from the baby's belly

3rd Stage of Labour

- Placenta separates from maternal uterine wall within three minutes of the birth of the child
- Leaves a raw bleeding area of about 7.5cm
- Myometrial function or the living ligatures control haemorrhage by squeezing blood vessels between myometrial strands

Active management of delivery of placenta

- Syntometrine 0.5mg with delivery of placenta
- Cord traction

Signs of placental separation

- A gush of blood may escape through the vagina
- The cord lengthens
- The height of the fundus rises

Placental delivery

Methods of placental delivery.

- **The Shultze method**
- The placenta slips through a hole in the membranes and the fetal side appears at the vulva with the membranes trailing behind like an inverted umbrella. Blood is contained in the inverted umbrella and should be carefully received into a container ready for measurement.
- **The Matthews Duncan(Dirty Duncan Method**)
- The placenta slides down sideways with the lateral border first like a button through a button hole. The maternal side is exposed and blood escapes

Examination of the placenta

The umbilical cord

- Extends from the fetal umbilicus to the fetal surface of the placenta.
- Composed of connective tissue and Wharton's jelly covered by the amnion.

- Has two arteries an extension of the hypogastric arteries.
- Umbilical arteries carry impure blood to the placenta
- A single artery is associated with other congenital abnormalities of the fetus.
- Umbilical vein contains pure blood from the placenta to the fetus.
- Hold the placenta by the cord so that the membranes hang like an inverted umbrella
- Note the type of cord insertion
- Note the length of the cord which should be about 56cms but cords can be shorter than this
- Note any true knots which cold be the cause of fetal distress and still birth
- Count the blood vessels in the cord
- Note any missing portions of the membranes as these are a source of post partum haemorrhage

- Note any blood vessels running to the edge of the membranes suggesting a succenturiate lobe which may cause haemorrhage and infection
- Note any holes in the membranes suggestive of a missing lobe
- Expose the maternal side and clean it with swab collecting any retro-placental clot and add to blood loss
- Inspect the cotyledons- absence of one suggestive of retained lobe, a source of post partum haemorrhage
- Take note of placental infarcts
- Weigh the placenta-it should be 1/6 of he baby's weight.

Before transferring the client to the postnatal ward:

- Inspect genital tract in good light for tears
- Repair the episiotomy and tears
- Check blood pressure and pulse

- Check height of fundus if high rub up a contraction to expel clots
- Check if infant is in good condition

26. OBSTRUCTED LABOUR

There is no advance of presenting part in the presence of good contractions.

The fault is in the passages and the passenger

Obstruction **commonly occurs at the inlet** but can take place at the outlet

Ideally obstructed labour should be avoided by careful palpation antenatally and before active labour so that the likely causes are dealt with appropriately.

Causes of Obstructed labour

- Contracted pelvis
- Malpresentation e.g shoulder presentation, compound presentation, brow, face
- Tumours e.g,. fibroids
- Large fetus(macrosomia)
- Fetalabnormalities e.g. hydrocephalus, double- headed monster, conjoined twins

Early Signs

- The presenting part remains floating despite good contractions
- The cervix dilates slowly and hangs loosely like an empty sleeve
- Membranes tend to rupture early

Late signs

- The uterus moulds around the fetus and does not relax between contractions
- The presenting part may become wedged or stuck in the pelvis
- Excessive moulding occurs
- A large caput forms
- Contractions may cease or a while and recommence with renewed vigour
- Bandl's ring may be seen abdominally around the umbilicus
- Maternal ketosis
- Fetal distress

Dangers to mother

- Rupture of uterus
- Haemorrhage
- Shock from haemorrhage, dehydration, exhaustion
- Vesico -vaginal fistula, recto-vaginal fistula
- Rupture of the bladder
- Death

Dangers to the fetus

- Fetal distress
- Intracranial haemorrhage
- Cerebral palsy
- Stillbirth
- Neonatal death

Prophylaxis

- Careful palpation antenatally to diagnose fetal abnormalities and refer clients for obstetric care early
- Careful monitoring of clients during labour to make early diagnosis of obstruction
- Lower segment caesarean section is done where diagnosis of likely obstruction is made

RUPTURE OF THE UTERUS

Causes

- Obstructed labour
- Trauma during difficult deliveries e.g. shoulder dystocia, after coming head of breech
- High doses of oxytocin
- Weak caesarean scar

Dangers of Ruptured Uterus

- Severe haemorrhage and shock
- Maternal death due to shock and haemorrhage

- Fetal loss

Warning signs of a rupture due to obstruction

- Tonic contractions
- Bandl's ring
- Signs of internal haemorrhage such as rapid pulse, restlessness, low blood pressure, sighing respirations
- Very tender lower abdomen
- Vaginal bleeding

Actual Rupture

- The woman may feel that something has given way
- Fetal distress followed by loss of fetal heart sounds
- The fetus can be palpated under the abdominal wall
- The woman may complain of shoulder pain a sign of blood in the peritoneum

- The uterus can be felt as a separate mass in the abdomen

Rupture of a weak caesarean scar

- Weak scar may be due to poor healing, pregnancy soon after previous caesarean section
- Rupture may occur during the last weeks of pregnancy due to over distension of abdomen in multiple pregnancy, polyhydramnios, big baby
- 'Silent rupture' may occur in the first stage of labour
- Rupture is gradual and incomplete and is usually over old scar
- Client complains of intermittent abdominal pain
- Severe abdominal pain and vomiting during labour

Management of clients with previous caesarean deliveries

- All clients with previous Caesarean deliveries must be referred in the third trimester for hospital delivery
- Oxytocin should not be used on clients with previous caesarean deliveries
- Abdominal palpation in clients with previous caesarean section must be minimal and gentle
- Complaints of abdominal pain or pain over the scar must be taken seriously and client must be prepared for Caesarean section immediately.
- Close observations for signs of shock and vaginal bleeding

General principles

- Aim at making early diagnosis of malpresentations and refer to obstetrician
- Oxytocin should not be given IM or orally as it is impossible to reverse or slow down its action.

Intrauterine Death

In the first trimester the various causes of abortion will cause intra- uterine death

In the middle trimester intrauterine death may be due to:

- Pre-eclampsia,
- Diabetes
- Fetal abnormalities,
- Ante-partum haemorrhage,
- Infections and infestations,
- Rhesus incompatibility

Signs of intra-uterine fetal death

- Abscence of fetal heart beat
- The mother does not feel fetal movements
- There is no uterine growth
- The height of fundus is small for dates
- There are no fetal heart sounds by Doppler
- Ultrasound scan shows Spalding's sign- gross overlapping of fetal skull bones

- Intra-fetal gas or bubbles of air can be seen in the lungs and heart of fetus
- The thoracic cage collapses
- There is hyper-flexion of the spine with abnormal fetal attitudes

Management

- Inform the couple of findings and likely management
- Labour is induced
- The fetus is usually macerated if death of the fetus occurred 12hours earlier
- The client is put on antibiotics post induction
- Investigation of possible causes must be done
- Family planning advice is given

Fresh Stillbirth

Causes: Hypoxia due to

- Placental insufficiency in pre-eclampsia, diabetes, renal disease, postmaturity

- True knots
- Abruption placenta
- Prematurity
- Prolonged labour
- Cord prolapse
- Difficult delivery

27. POST MATURITY

This is when pregnancy goes beyond 42 weeks

Management

- Ascertain pregnancy dates by going back to the pregnancy dates
- Induction of labour
- Episiotomy and assisted delivery since the head does not mould
- Caesarean section may be done to prevent prolonged labour and fetal distress

Risks of post maturity

- Perinatal mortality is high
- Placental insufficiency is common
- Stillbirth is common
- Cervical,vaginal and perineal tears

The postmature baby

- Has hard skull bones, mall fontanelles and narrow sutures

- The skin is dry and peeling off
- There is no subcutaneous fat
- Nails are long

28. CAESAREAN SECTION

Delivery of a baby through a surgical operation on the abdomen is called Caesarean Section.

Elective Caesarean section is planned in advance where reasons why a woman cannot have a normal delivery have been identified.

Emergency Caesarean section in which there is a sudden turn of events in the progress of labour in the condition of the mother or baby that requires that urgent action be taken to save lives.

Types of Caesarean Section

Lower segment caesarean section or Pfannestiel incision is transverse just above symphysis pubis

- It heals well and the scar may not be obvious
- Makes early ambulation easy
- Does not interfere with sitting and breast feeding

Classical Caesarean section

- An incision extending from above the symphysis pubis to the umbilicus or just above
- Uterine incision extends to the upper segment
- Very uncomfortable when client tries to sit
- Uncomfortable when breastfeeding
- Slow in healing and limits client's activity post delivery

Indications for a Caesarean Section

Caesarean Section is done to save the lives of both mother and baby.

Maternal Causes

- **Severe Pre-eclampsia and eclampsia** requires that the woman is delivered as soon as possible through Caesarean Section.
- **Abnormal uterine action**. A woman may have very weak contractions that cause

labour to be prolonged. A caesarean section is necessary to deliver the woman before complications arise.

- **Contracted pelvis**
- **Cephalo pelvic disproportion**
- Previous Caesarean section
- Abruption placentae
- Placenta praevia

Caesarean Section can be done to save a baby .

- Where the baby is large (macrosomia) such as in diabetes and potential diabetes

In abnormal presentations such as:

- Transverse Lie.
- Compound Presentation **likely to cause obstructed labour. It is** impossible for the baby to pass through the birth canal.
- Large Breech Presentation. A small baby as in premature labour may negotiate his way through the pelvis

- Shoulder dystocia
- Abnormal fetus e.g. hydrocephalus, conjoined twins
- Locked twins
- Retained twin
- **Fetal distress characterised by Meconeum stained liquor or fetal tarchycardia or bradycardia.** The baby must be delivered quickly
- **Cord Prolapse and cord presentation.** This usually occurs when the membranes break and the presenting part does not fit snugly against the cervix. The cord may be compressed against the presenting part and the bony pelvis as the baby negotiates his way out and may go into spasms interfering with the baby's breathing.

Women should be advised to deliver in health institutions where help is readily available.

Care after Caesarean Section

- Post operative observations must be done strictly
- Vital signs such as Blood pressure and pulse
- Look out for bleeding from wound and signs of internal haemorrhage
- Pain relief must be given according to client's needs
- The client must be assisted in finding comfortable breast feeding position

Advice to clients

- Advise clients that It is normal to feel tired in the first 48hours after an operation.
- With an epidural their activity is curtailed for the first eight hours. Encourage leg movements to prevent deep vein thrombosis and deep breathing exercises to prevent chest complications as soon as possible.

- Clients must be advised to look after the suture line (caesarean scar) well. Avoiding water over it until it is completely dry.
- Advise clients to report to the midwives for advice the presence of a raw patch or discharge from wound.
- Clients must be advised to avoid strenuous activity and allow the body time to recover and the wound time to heal.
- A nutritious diet rich in fruit and vegetables must be advised.
- Clients must be advised to wait for at least two years before another pregnancy to allow the abdominal muscles to heal.

29. POST PARTUM HAEMORRHAGE

- Haemorrhage is one of the leading causes of maternal mortality in the world
- Haemorrhage exposes women to morbidity and mortality by the nature of its severity and especially where skills in managing it are lacking.
- Blood loss of more than 600mls after delivery of a baby is termed **Postpartum haemorrhage**

Primary post partum haemorrhage within first 24 hours post delivery due to:

- Failure of effective uterine contraction caused by uterine atony common in:
- multiparous women,
- multiple pregnancy,
- hydatidiform mole
- fibroids
- prolonged labour
- following general anaesthesia

- Retention of placental tissue
- Antepartum haemorrhage especially abruption placenta and placenta praevia and release of retroplacental clot
- Clotting defects such as hypofibrinogenaemia and low platlets and other blood discrasias
- Trauma such as ruptured uterus or torn cervix or vaginal wall lacerations
- If bleeding occurs before expulsion of placenta an attempt to expel the placenta must be made by rubbing up a contraction and use cord traction to deliver the placenta

Secondary post partum haemorrhage after 24hours due to

- Retained membranes or placental cotyledon
- Dislogded clot
- Infection such as myometritis
- Onset of choriocarcinoma

Signs of severe blood loss are:

- Restlessness followed by severe weakness
- Rapid thready pulse and low blood pressure.
- Parlour of skin which is easily noticed in the mucosa of the mouth, the tongue, palms and nail beds in dark skinned people and on the face in light skinned people.
- Breathlessness and sighing respirations
- The skin may become cold and clammy
- The client may faint or collapse

Principles of managing haemorrhage:

- Replace lost fluids by the use of an intravenous line.
- Quickly identify source of the haemorrhage and manage

In Abortion

- Evacuation of uterus to remove retained products of conception

- An oxytocic drug may be needed
- Infection must be treated with antibiotics
- Haemoglobin level must be assessed and haemoglobin supplements such as iron and vitamins given

Antenatal haemorrhage

- Replace fluids to prevent shock
- Quickly identify source of haemorrhage
- Allay anxiety
- Inspect the tone of the uterus.
- Inspect the birth canal for hidden tears and suturing of the tears must be done immediately.
- Rub up a contraction and administer an oxytocic drug immediately if the cause of haemorrhage is uterine atony.

The loss of lives can be avoided by close monitoring of the women and immediate transfer of women to facilities with adequate resources for resuscitation.

Observations

- Blood pressure and pulse must be monitored every half hour for the first two hours, every hour for the following four hours and two hourly for four hours then four hourly thereafter for the first 24hours

- Blood pressure and pulse should be checked before transferring a mother into the postnatal ward and continued hourly for four hours then thereafter four hourly throughout the stay in the health facility until the woman is discharged home.

- Pad checks should be done hourly in the first two hours post delivery, then two hourly for four hours then four hourly thereafter.

- Close monitoring should be continued until the postnatal mother feels strong enough to be discharged from the unit.

Fundal Height

- The height of fundus may rise where there is internal bleeding due to atony of the uterus.

- Contract the uterus by 'rubbing up a contraction' to activate the uterine muscle to contract or giving an oxytoxic drug.
- Fundal height measurement and uterine consistency should be observed hourly for four hours post delivery especially in clients likely to have postpartum haemorrhage such is multiparous clients, clients who have had difficult prolonged labour, clients who have had multiple deliveries and clients who have had surgical deliveries.
- Immediately post delivery, the consistency of the contracted uterus must feel like a tennis ball.
- A soft boggy or dough-like uterus is a sign of poor contraction of the uterus
- Take immediate action to assist the uterus to contract using current measures according to management policy.
- After delivery, the height of the fundus is below the umbilicus and should continue to

decrease until the uterus is no longer palpable around fourteen days post delivery.

- The fundal height should be measured on a day-to-day basis and should decrease by approximately one centimetre a day post delivery.

Perineal Care

- Clients are advised to wash the perineum clean with each change of sanitary towel or every two hours to avoid odours and to promote healing.

Prevention of Anaemia

- All women should have their haemoglobin checked before discharge from the postnatal ward.
- Anaemia affects involution and delays repair of tissues post delivery.
- Women who have lost a lot of blood are generally lethargic, frail and tend to have a slow recovery post delivery.

- Anaemia causes debilitation in women post delivery and exposes them to heart failure and infections that may interfere with successful breast feeding, self-care and baby care.

Bladder Care.

The client must be encouraged to empty her bladder two hourly initially then four hourly to prevent over-distension of the bladder which interferes with uterine contraction and successful involution.

- The postnatal mother must be encouraged to take plenty of fluids to encourage the bladder to empty frequently by so doing regaining its tone.
- It is important to observe for hesitancy to empty the bladder and retention of urine which may occur where a woman has perineal trauma.
- Complaints of dysuria must be taken seriously and the woman should be tested

for urinary tract infection. Dysuria is associated with poor asceptic technique during labour and perineal repair, too many vaginal examinations, and inadequate treatment of urinary tract infection in pregnancy.

- Urine retention post delivery is associated with damage to nerves and hypotonic pelvic musculature
- Perineal hygiene that emphasizes washing and wiping the perineal area from front backwards and change of pads two hourly and when the pad is soaked should be encouraged.
- Use of clean pads should be encouraged to prevent infection.

Ambulation

- Early ambulation post delivery is advised to prevent thrombo-embolic and chest complications

- Passive exercises and movement in bed must be encouraged for those women who must stay in bed for long periods because their conditions do not allow them to get out of bed early.
- Encourage deep breathing exercises immediately post delivery to promote cardio-respiratory fitness and to encourage expulsion of lochia.

30. THE NEWBORN

- Ensure that the baby cries at birth.
- Assess Apgar Score at 1,5,and 10 minutes of birth

Apgar score

Baby's Condition	0	1	2	1min	5min	10min
Activity (muscle tone)	Limp/Flaccid	Weak	Active			
Pulse/Heart rate	Absent	Bradycardia	Normal			
Response to stimuli Grimace, reflex, irritability	Absent	Weak	Active			
Appearance(skin colour)	Grey	Dusky	Pink			
Respiration	Absent	Rib recession Gasping	Normal			
Total score						

- Clear airways by soft suction.

- Hold the baby head lower than the legs so that liquor flows out.

- A good cry expands the lungs and establishes good respiration and normal circulation.

- The baby may need oxygen by face mask if there are signs of cyanosis

- Wipe baby dry and drape warmly to prevent hypothermia.

- A quick examination of the newborn must be done as soon as the baby is born.

- Thorough examination should be done after the baby has settled post delivery within the first 24hours, before the baby is discharged from hospital, on the first domiciliary visit and at six weeks post delivery. For details of examination of the newborn, see the book 'Post Natal Care.'

Examine for Normalcy from head to toe

The size and shape of the head to exclude hydrocephalus and microcephally

Hydrocephaly

- The head is unusually big because of blockage of the flow of cerebro-spinal fluid
- The sutures and fontanelles are large
- The skull bones are thinned out and feel soft on palpation

- The face is small
- The forehead is prominent and the eyes are small
- Usually adopts the breech presentation but where the presentation is cephalic, the head remains high ad will not engage in the pelvis
- The wide sutures can be felt on palpation
- Labour will be obstructed

- In breech presentation labour is obstructed as the baby is born as far as the umbilicus

Management

- The midwife must do a careful palpation to make an early diagnosis
- Refer for verification of diagnosis if unsure
- In early diagnosis, a therapeutic abortion is done
- In late diagnosis, a caesarean section is performed
- In obstructed labour a craniotomy is done

Encephalocele

This is a tumour of the brain covered with meninges and protrudes through the lambda or the sutures

- Depending on the size they may obstruct labour
- An encephalocele contains brain substance
- It is opaque
- It does not fluctuate

213

- Usually has a pedicle

A meningocele

- Contains cerebro-spinal fluid
- Is fluctuant
- Does not pulsate
- Becomes tense when the baby cries
- May rupture during labour otherwise it is corrected surgically

Anencephally

A severe derformity common in female fetus

- The vault of the skull and cerebellum are absentMay be accompanied by spina bifida
- Polyhydramnios usually present in pregnancy
- Increased levels of alphafetoproteins in amniotic fluid in early pregnancy
- Labour is induced prematurely
- Labour can be prolonged to allow for passage of shoulders

- May live for a few minutes
- Reassure mother that subsequent babies are likely to be normal
- Advise to book for care early

Spina Bifida

- Failure of the neural arches of the vertebrae to unite causing the meninges and sometimes the spinal cord to protrude
- Cover the open wound with sterile dressing and refer
- Mild cases are corrected by surgery

Observe for trauma and signs of intracranial injury in likely excessive compression of the head for first 24hours in:

- contracted pelvis,
- large baby,
- occipito-posterior positions,
- breech,
- precipitate labour

- prolonged labour
- preterm labour
- face to pubes

Exclude birth injuries such as **cephalhaematoma** and **caput succedaneum**, **haematoma** and **intracranial** injury.

Caput succedaneum

- Due to pressure of cervix on presenting part
- Venous blood is retarded
- Presenting part becomes congested and oedematous
- May occur in prolonged labour such as occipito-posterior
- Ocassionally if the head is held for long on the perineum
- Is present at birth
- Pits on pressure
- May cross a suture
- Reduces in size with time
- Should disappear within 36hours

- It is always unilateral

Cephalhaematoma

- Swelling on the fetal skull
- It is effusion of blood under the periosteum
- Caused by friction between the fetal skull and pelvis and
- Excessive moulding

Occurs commonly in:

- Cephalopelvic disproprtion

Quick delivery of the head such as in:

- Precipitate labour
- After coming head of breech

Characteristics:

- Appears after 12hours of childbirth
- Does not cross a suture
- Grows larger as bleeding occurs
- May persist for two weeks or more

- It is firm and does not pit on pressure
- Can be bilateral
- Give Vit. K1
- Refer for haemoglobin estimation

Common fractures in newborn

- Indentations may occur on skull showing compression against promontory of the sacrum
- Fracture of the humerus may occur in breech delivery and shoulder presentation
- Fractures of Femur also common in breech delivery
- Fracture of the spine is rare

Facial palsy

- Common in forceps delivery where the 7th cranial nerve may be pinched during delivery of the head.
- One side of the mouth droops and milk may dribble during feeding

- The eye on the affected side remains open
- Corrects itself after a few weeks

The neck may be twisted in breech delivery and shoulder dystocia

Erb's paralysis or waiter's tip arm

This is injury to the brachial plexus under the clavicle. Common in breech delivery but can occur in vertex delivery.

Extra Digits

These are fairly common and are usually attaché by loose skin.

- Black Silk can be used to tie them off and usually drop off within a week
- Refer where there is evidence of bone attachment

Injury to internal organs especially the liver can also occur in breech delivery. Suspect internal injury where the baby turns grey and collapse.

Cleft lip and palate

- This is lack of union of the fronto-nasal palate.
- A baby may have just a cleft lip or may have both cleft lip and palate
- These deformities may be unilateral or bilateral pausing a real challenge in feeding the baby. Milk flows out in cleft lip. The mother must be encouraged to exercise a lot of patience.

Refer for surgery.

- Feeding problems are more serious in cleft palate where cyanosis can occur as milk flows into the respiratory system.
- The baby can be fitted with dental plates especially in bilateral cleft lip and palate changed periodically as baby grows until surgery is performed
- Expressed milk can be given using a large special teat or a spoon.

Exclude oesophageal atresia especially in babies whose mothers had polyhydramnios.

- Suspect oesophageal atresia where baby frothes from the mouth and nostrils on first feed.
- Insert a fine nasogastric tube and it will not go down. Refer immediately for surgery.

Duodenal Atresia

- The baby vomits milk followed by bile characterized by green vomitus
- The baby's abdomen may be distended
- Refer for surgery immediately
- The baby is put on IV fluids and food is witheld until after surgery.

Exomphalos

This is when abdominal contents are outside the abdominal wall.

- Contents contained in a thin sac of the peritoneum that escapes from the abdomen through a large opening on the umbilicus.
- Cover with paraffin gauze or a sterile towel
- Transfer for surgery immediately.

Pyloric stenosis

- Baby has projectile vomiting of mucus is noted
- Waves of peristalsis can be noted on the abdomen after feeds
- Usually noticed after the first week
- **Refer for surgery**

Umbilical hernia

A swelling around the umbilicus noted after the umbilical cord has dropped off.

- May resolve itself if small
- Refer large hernias for surgical opinion.

Check for the anal patency by inserting a rectal thermometer

Amelia (no arms) and Phocomelia (abscence of long bones)

Such conditions although rare do occur due to drugs taken in the first trimester

- The parents with babies with congenital abnormalities need constant support and reassurance.
- Health personnel must advise clients against off the counter drugs in pregnancy
- Health personnel must always ask women if they are pregnant before prescribing drugs.
- Reassure parents and inform them about prosthesis
- Refer them to access relevant services

Club Foot

Talipes Equino Varus

The foot is bent downwards and inwards

- May be unilateral(one foot) or bilateral (both feet)
- The cause is not known but associated with oligohydramnios and tumours like fibroids
- To correct the deformity, splinting and application of Plaster of Paris is done from the first day post delivery
- Surgery may be necessary in extreme cases

Talipes Calcaneo-Valgus

The foot is turned outwards, the opposite of Talipes Equino Varus.

- The deformity is considered less serious than Equino Varus
- Correction is by splinting and application of Plaster Of Paris

Achondroplasia

- The baby is born with short limbs
- The body is of normal length
- Long bones fail to develop in early fetal life.

- Majority of the babies survive and have normal mental development
- They become dwarfs
- It is important to inform the mother of the baby's prognosis and reassure her.
- It is also important to link the parents with other parents with children with the same condition.
- Refer parents to associations and organizations with interest in the condition

Mongolism/ Down's syndrome (Trisomy 21)

Mongols have an extra chromosome giving them 47 chromosomes instead of 46

The condition is associated with maternal ageing and is significant in mothers over the age of 35

Characteristics of a mongul

- Small head with flat occiput
- Low set ears
- Upward slanting eyes

- Small mouth and large tongue
- Short hands
- An unbroken palmer crease from side to side(the simian crease)
- The big toe is widely separated from the rest of the toes
- May have cardiac lesion
- Parents must be reassured as Mongols may be slow learners, may be slow to talk and may not have a clear speech but are happy children.
- **Inform parents about facilities available**

Reflexes

The baby's reaction to various tests must be checked to assess for alertness and normalcy in the baby.

The Rooting Reflex

This is testing for the baby's reaction to suckling reflexes. A finger gently moved on the cheeks from the angles of the mouth should make the baby turn his head towards the finger and make sucking movements.

The Walking /Stepping Reflex

When baby is put on his feet, he attempts to lift his foot to walk. Failure to lift legs shows weakness and probable injury of the nerves of the legs which is more likely in difficult breech delivery.

Moro Reflex

When a baby is suddenly lowered down, he panics, and suddenly extends and abducts his limbs. Birth injuries involving nerves may be identified by observing the reaction of the limbs.

The Grasp Reflex

If a finger is placed in the newborn's hand, the baby grasps the finger tightly so much that it is possible to test for traction and muscle tone. Weak grasp or failure to grasp the finger is an indication of weakness mostly due to injury of the radial or ulna nerves. The baby must be referred to neuro-specialists.

Asymmetrical Tonic Neck Reflex

When the baby's neck is passively turned to the side, the limbs on the same side to which the neck is turned are extended while those on the opposite side are flexed. This is suggestive of neck injury at birth especially after breech delivery and shoulder dystocia.

Glabellar Reflex

When the root or the nose is gently tapped, the eyes are screwed. The responsiveness of the baby to the reflexes is an indication of the alertness or passivity of the baby.

31.BREAST FEEDING

Breast milk is the natural baby's milk, and contains immune bodies to prevent infections in the baby

Breast milk is available all the time. The mother must be encouraged to drink fluids to encourage an increased flow.

Breast milk is always at the right temperature so it does not need warming

Breast milk is nutritious with all food values in the correct proportions

Breast milk is whole; there is no need for additives

Breast milk is environment friendly, it does not create litter in its production and after use

Breast milk is easily stored and cannot be contaminated by dust or any environmental wastes as it is within the mother

Breast milk is economical, there are no expenses incurred to acquire it

Breast milk promotes close relationships between mother and baby

The importance of a nutritious diet and taking plenty of fluids to improve the flow of milk should be emphasized.

About the Author

Nester Kadzviti Murira studied for her PhD at Birmingham City University, UK, School of Health and Social Care Research. She has a Masters Degree in Medical Education from University of Dundee, Scotland, Centre for Medical Education. She has a B.Ed.Adult Education, and Diploma in Adult and Nursing Education from the University of Zimbabwe. She has a Diploma in Midwifery and General Nursing from Zimbabwe.

Nester has worked as a Health Care Training Consultant, a Lecturer in Reproductive Health, a Midwifery Tutor, a Research Midwife,a Maternity Home manager, and a Domiciliary Postnatal Services Care manager in Zimbabwe. Nester has worked in several Primary Care Trusts in UK.

She is a published researcher and author of health books, children's books and contemporary subjects.

www.ingramcontent.com/pod-product-compliance
Lightning Source LLC
Chambersburg PA
CBHW070853180526
45168CB00005B/1796